UNDERSTANDING THE BODY ORGANS

&

THE EIGHT LAWS OF HEALTH

Compiled by
Celeste Lee

TEACH Services, Inc.
Brushton, New York

© 1992 by Abundant Life Ministry
© 1997 by TEACH Services, Inc.
ISBN 0-945383-44-4
LOC 94-60068

Published by:

TEACH Services, Inc.
RR 1, Box 182
Brushton, New York 12916 USA

Table of Contents

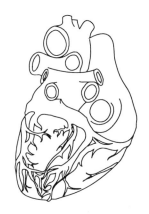

THE HEART

The heart is the main organ of the circulatory system. It is located in the chest cavity, nestled between the lungs and protected by the breast bone and the ribs.

The heart is an involuntary muscle. It is also a strong and specialized muscle. The heart is about the size of a person's fist and the average weight is 10 to 11 ounces. It is divided into four chambers, two on the left side and two on the right side. One chamber on each side to pull the blood into the heart and one chamber on each side to push the blood through the arteries.

The purpose of the heart is to pump enough blood at high enough pressure to constantly circulate the blood to all parts of the body. The right side of the heart pumps the blood to the lungs, where the blood releases carbon dioxide and picks up oxygen. The blood returns to the left side of the heart where it is pumped to the entire body. Throughout the body the blood delivers nutrients, oxygen, and hormones to the cells, and carries the waste products to disposal sites such as the liver, lungs, and kidneys.

Some interesting facts about the heart are:

1) It pumps about 1,250 gallons of blood daily.
2) At each beat the heart exerts about eight pounds of pressure on the circulatory system. This amounts to about 30,000 pounds per hour.
3) It works nine hours in the twenty-four hour day and rests fifteen.

"Day by day the heart throbs, doing its regular appointed task, unceasingly forcing its crimson current to all parts of the body." *Life Sketches*, p. 87.

"Keep thy heart with all diligence; for out of it are the issues of life." *Proverbs* 4:23. The word issues that is used here means "sources". This is true in the physical as well as the spiritual aspect of life.

Benefits of exercise

Since the heart is a muscle it must be kept in condition by exercise, preferably every day. Exercise that benefits the heart is called "cardiopulmonary" exercise, (cardio = heart, pulmonary = lungs). To receive the full benefits of cardiopulmonary exercise, one needs to exercise continually for 20 minutes every day. The benefits to the heart from this kind of daily exercise are:

1) Increase stroke volume, the amount of blood pumped with each heart beat.

2) Decrease pulse rate, thereby giving the heart more time to rest between beats.

Diet

There is also another important factor in regaining and maintaining a healthy heart. THE DIET! The heart as a muscle pumps the blood cells throughout the entire body. The bloodstream is used as a network of roads, taking what is put in the system to all the body. If the arteries become clogged, because of an improper diet, the heart must pump harder to maintain circulation. Therefore, what is eaten has a direct effect on the heart. Three things that greatly affect the health of the heart that are completely controlled by the diet are:

1) cholesterol,

2) fats in the blood known as triglycerides,

3) and the most important of these three, dangerous saturated fats.

Cholesterol

Cholesterol is a thick, waxy substance which acts like wet cement in the bloodstream. This settles on the lining of the arteries and slowly builds up resulting in hardening of the arteries. The body makes a cholesterol which is beneficial to the system. But the low density lipoprotein cholesterol (LDL-C) is harmful and responsible for heart attacks. This harmful cholesterol comes only from animal products. All food that does not contain any animal product contains no cholesterol.

The amount of fats in the blood (triglycerides) is another important factor in maintaining a healthy heart. These triglycerides tend to cause the platelet and red blood cells to be sticky and to clump together decreasing the flow of oxygen. Saturated fats are those fats which raise the level of cholesterol in the blood and cause the body to retain more cholesterol when animal products are a part of the diet. For this reason saturated fats are exceptionally harmful. If the system only contains the cholesterol produced by the body, the intake of saturated fats will not be a problem, as they cannot cause hardening of the arteries without the presence of animal cholesterol.

Saturated fats

When meat is taken into the system it causes several reactions concerning cholesterol. The cholesterol it contains is added to the system and as the meat is full of saturated fat it will cause the body to retain more cholesterol. This is done by the lack of fiber in meat which results in a build up of bile acids in the bowel. These bile acids must be promptly eliminated or they are recycled and trigger still higher levels of blood cholesterol.

Meat and cholesterol

There are two very common factors that also produce higher triglyceride levels in the blood stream. Refined sugar in the diet will greatly increase the triglyceride level in the blood. The other one is eating between meals which causes a flooding of the blood stream with triglycerides. No wonder we are told, "Never should a morsel of food pass the lips between meals." *Counsels on Health*, p. 118.

Other factors

"Especially harmful are the custards and puddings in which milk, eggs, and sugar are the chief ingredients." *Ministry of Healing*, p. 302. Why? Milk and cream contain a high level of saturated fats which cause cholesterol levels in the blood to rise. Second, sugar raises the triglycerides, blood fats, to a higher level. Lastly, animal cholesterol is highly concentrated in eggs. A large egg contains 250 milligrams of cholesterol, plus a large amount of saturated fat. When all three are present together blood cholesterol is elevated more rapidly than by one of them alone.

Clearly, we can see why God's people are to return to the original diet of fruits, nuts, grains, and vegetables, (*Genesis* 1:29; 3:18) just from the effect that eating these things have in maintaining a healthy heart.

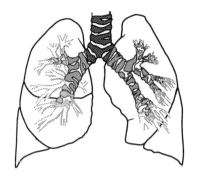

THE LUNGS

The lungs are the major part of the respiratory system. The respiratory system works closely with the circulatory system. The lungs are located between the spine in the back, and the chest bone and ribs in the front.

The two lungs are soft, spongy, and very elastic. They weigh just over a pound each. Each lung is surrounded by an airtight covering called the pleura. There are three lobes in the right lung and only two in the left. If one of the lobes becomes damaged the others continue to function.

Purpose

The lungs purpose is to supply oxygen to the body and to release the carbon dioxide, which is a waste gas. The process of exchange is done in the alveoli, which are very tiny air sacs. They are surrounded by capillaries with only very thin walls separating them. Oxygen molecules seep through these walls to the blood cells. At the same time the carbon dioxide is released into the lung to be expelled.

Since the lungs have no muscles, the muscles around the chest cavity do the work. The biggest worker in breathing is the diaphragm. It is a sheet of muscle connected to the backbone and the front of the rib cage. In slow breathing it only moves an inch or less, but during vigorous exercise it can move up and down several inches.

Interesting facts

Some interesting facts about the lungs are:

1) They hold three quarts of air.

2) The lungs discharge 30 quarts of carbonic acid per hour through the breath.

3) Five quarts of blood pass through the lungs every minute.

4) The air sacs of the lungs, if flattened into a sheet, would contain 1,100 square feet.

5) The average adult lungs inhale and exhale about 20,000 times a day.

Benefits of exercise

Even though the lungs are not muscles they benefit from exercise. "Cardiopulmonary" exercise, (cardio = heart, pulmonary = lungs) is recommended as the best for the heart and lungs. To obtain the benefits of this exercise you must exercise continually for 20 minutes. This exercise, which causes increased breathing through the lungs, benefits not only the respiratory system, but the entire body. Some of the benefits resulting from this are:

1) Full, deep intakes of pure air purify the blood.

2) Oxygen electrifies the whole system.

3) Good respiration soothes the nerves, stimulates the appetite, helps in digestion and induces a good sleep.

4) Exercise strengthens the lungs to perform their work properly.

Proper breathing

"In order to have good blood, we must breathe well...The lungs should be allowed the greatest freedom possible. Their capacity is developed by free action; it diminishes if they are cramped and compressed. Hence the ill effects of the practice so common, especially in sedentary pursuits, of stooping at one's work. In this position it is impossible to breathe deeply. Superficial breathing soon becomes a habit, and the lungs lose their power to expand. A similar effect is produced by tight lacing. Sufficient room is not given to the lower part of the chest; the abdominal muscles, which were designed to aid in breathing, do not have full play, and the lungs are restricted in their action.

Results of insufficient oxygen

"Thus an insufficient supply of oxygen is received. The blood moves sluggishly. The waste, poisonous matter, which should be thrown off in the exhalations from the lungs, is retained, and the blood becomes impure. Not only the lungs, but the stomach, liver, and the brain are affected. The skin becomes sallow, digestion is retarded; the heart is depressed; the brain is clouded; the thoughts are confused; gloom settles upon the spirits; the whole system becomes depressed and inactive, and peculiarly susceptible to disease.

"The lungs are constantly throwing off impurities, and they need to be constantly supplied with fresh air. Impure air does not afford the necessary supply of oxygen, and the blood passes to the brain and other organs without being vitalized. Hence the necessity of thorough ventilation. To live in close, ill ventilated rooms, where the air is dead and vitiated, weakens the entire system. It becomes peculiarly sensitive to the influence of cold, and a slight exposure induces disease. It is close confinement indoors that makes many women pale and feeble. They breathe the same air over and over until it becomes laden with poisonous matter thrown off through the lungs and pores, and impurities are thus conveyed back to the lungs." *Ministry of Healing*, p. 272–274.

Fresh oxygen necessary

Water is also important to the health of the lungs. The lungs are made up of 75% water. Since the lungs are an eliminating organ the water in them needs to be fresh to keep them clean. The lungs release a minimum of one pint of water in the exhaled breath every day. If there is not enough water for the kidneys to do their job of elimination some of the waste is eliminated through the lungs, which adds to the work they must do.

Importance of water

The lungs need fresh, pure air 24 hours a day to do their work of supplying oxygen to the red blood cells. It is easy to understand that neglecting to provide the lungs with fresh, pure air causes many problems for the whole system. God has so lovingly given us pure air to maintain and restore our health. Let us do our part to give the lungs what they need to supply the whole body so we may have health in abundance.

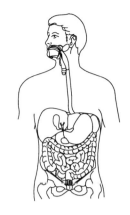

THE DIGESTIVE SYSTEM

The digestive system of the body involves several organs and is quite complex. The system of digestion starts in the mouth and continues for 27 to 30 feet, in a normal adult, to the anus. The 30 feet of tube is called the alimentary canal. It includes the mouth, esophagus, stomach, duodenum, the small intestine, and the colon which is also called the large intestine. The liver and pancreas aid in digestion but are not part of the alimentary canal.

Digestive system is complex

The purpose of digestion is to take the food that is eaten and break it down into nutrients—basic materials the body can use. The food eaten can be classified into groups of nutrients such as: starch, sugar, fat, protein, minerals and vitamins. These must pass through the four digestive juices—the saliva, gastric juice, pancreatic juice and the bile, in order to be prepared for absorption into the blood stream to be used by the cells. During a lifetime the digestion system processes between 60,000 and 100,000 pounds of food.

Purpose

There are three classes of foods that the body needs to maintain its proper functions.

Three essential classes of food

CLASS ONE—Heat and Energy Foods

Class one

STARCH	*SUGAR*
Cereals	Sugar
Breads	Maple sugar
Macaroni	Sorghum
Tapioca	Honey
Certain vegetables	Sweet fruits

FATS
Olives
Vegetable oils
Salad oils
Nuts
Soy beans
Milk

Class two

CLASS TWO—Building and Repair Food

PROTEIN

Grains	Beans
Soybeans	Lentils
Peas	Nuts

Class three

CLASS THREE—Regulators of Body Processes

WATER	*MINERALS*
Pure fruit or	Bran of cereals
vegetable juices	Vegetables
Fruit	Legumes
Vegetables	Fruits
	Nuts

CELLULOSE	*VITAMINS*
Indigestible matter	The vital spark
Bran	which activates the
Framework of fruits	other food elements,
and vegetables	without which growth
	cannot occur or
	continue.

Proper balance needed

Most people overeat from Class One—too much starch and sugar. Also, the need for protein, which is the building food, is not as great as is usually eaten. The average person does not get enough water, minerals and vitamins. The result is that the system becomes clogged with starch, sugar, fat and protein which cannot be properly utilized without water, minerals, and vitamins.

Mouth—start of digestion

In this lesson we will look at the very first place digestion begins—the mouth. The mouth is composed of the teeth, tongue, hard palate, soft palate and salivary glands. Each of these has its own part to play to ensure digestion is started properly.

When food is taken into the mouth the teeth begin their work of breaking it up and mixing it with the saliva. The chewing of food starts the whole digestive system functioning. Chewing the food thoroughly is very important for several reasons.

1) It starts the saliva flowing freely and causes the gastric and other digestive juices to begin to flow.

2) It causes the peristaltic waves to begin. These waves move the food through the alimentary canal.

3) The longer the food is chewed the more completely the starch is digested. This is done by the saliva which contains a starch-digesting ferment.

4) The nerves of taste, through the tasting of the food, thoroughly regulate the amount of food the body needs. Overeating is often a result of hasty eating.

5) Proper chewing gives the teeth the exercise they need to be preserved properly.

Saliva is produced by salivary glands in the mouth and cheeks. Saliva is colorless and watery in appearance. Saliva contains ptyalin an enzyme which changes starches into simple sugar. It also produces an alkaline (acid-neutralizing) chemical reaction. There is also some mucus in saliva which lubricates the food that is chewed so that it may be swallowed.

Some interesting facts concerning saliva are:

1) Six salivary glands supply about three pints of saliva daily.

2) Saliva is made up of the following: potassium 49%, sodium 9%, iron oxide 5%, sulphur 6%, phosphorus 18%, and chlorine 17%.

It is necessary to have enough of the above mentioned minerals in the diet to maintain the digesting ability of the saliva.

There are, at the back of the tongue, nerves of taste. These nerves, when brought into contact with finely dissolved particles of food, send a message to the nerve center in the brain, that tells the gastric glands of the stomach to produce digestive juices. Various flavors in natural foods stimulate these nerves to produce the proper quantity and quality of gastric juices necessary to digest the particular food being eaten.

When the process of digestion that starts in the mouth is understood, the harm caused by chewing gum is easy to see. When the taste nerves are stimulated by chewing gum they send a message to the brain to release gastric juices into the stomach. When no food travels down the alimentary canal to the stomach to be digested, these juices remain in the stomach, resulting in too much acid in the stomach. (To much acid in the stomach will be discussed in the next lesson.)

Saliva alkaline

As mentioned before, the saliva is made up of mostly minerals. All the digestive fluids are alkaline except the gastric juice, which is an acid. Again a proper balance of these four digestive fluids is essential to the proper digestion of food. Salvia is alkaline. To keep its proper alkaline balance a person needs to eat 75% of the their total food intake from the alkaline food group. (See appendix for alkaline/acid food chart.) This food group is found in the greatest concentration in Class Three. It is important for digestion as well as other bodily functions, that we eat of the best food that can give the system the nutrients it needs most.

In the next lesson we will continue with the digestive process following the food through the alimentary canal from the mouth to the stomach. We will see how food relates to the acid and alkaline fluids in the body.

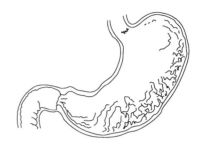

THE STOMACH

In this lesson we continue the digestion process that has started in the mouth. After the food has been thoroughly chewed it passes down the esophagus to the stomach. This is done by the contracting of the muscular walls of the esophagus, causing the food to be transported to the stomach. At the top of the stomach is a sphincter muscle which, when open allows food to enter and when closed keeps the contents of the stomach from returning into the esophagus.

Location and size of the stomach

The stomach is located under the diaphragm on the left side of the abdomen. It is protected by the five lower ribs. The stomach is a kind of elastic bag, which can expand to hold 2 1/4 pints or approximately 5 cups of food or water.

The stomach's purpose is to digest the protein that is eaten. We learned in the last lesson that the starch is digested in the mouth. The stomach continues the breakdown of starch started in the mouth with the salvia, and starts the breakdown of protein so the small intestine may do the largest amount of digestion and absorption. As the digestion process continues we will learn how other organs do their part of digesting and absorbing certain foods.

Purpose

The stomach is surrounded by muscles that are lengthwise, circular and oblique (slanted). These muscles work in waves to churn the food with the gastric juices. These waves pass along the stomach at the rate of three to five waves per minute. At the bottom of the stomach is another sphincter muscle, called the pylorus, which controls the release of food into the small intestine where it is more completely digested.

Stomach muscles

There are approximately thirty-five million glands in the stomach that release one to two quarts of gastric juice daily to dissolve the protein elements of the food. Other glands release mucus which forms a protective layer in the stomach so the acid from the gastric juice does not burn the stomach wall.

Balance of gastric juices

As mentioned in the last lesson the gastric juice is the only one of the four digestive juices that is acid based. If the gastric juices are too high or too low in acid it will cause problems in the stomach and thus interfere with the digestion process. Too much acid in the stomach results from the glands being over stimulated so that the gastric juice contains too much hydrochloric acid. This is what digests protein and when there is too much hydrochloric acid it will start to attack the stomach which is made of protein. It results in a burning sensation and heartburn may be the result. A high content of hydrochloric acid will also cause the muscle at the top of the stomach to relax and cause acid and food to be forced through the esophagus into the mouth. Normal gastric juice is .2 of 1% hydrochloric acid. When an excess of protein is eaten, it creates the need for more hydrochloric acid, raising the level to .3–.6 of 1%.

Alkaline diet

The most important way to correct to much hydrochloric acid in the stomach is to eat a high alkaline diet. The worse the condition is the more fiber should be removed from the diet to allow for healing. Fat foods such as olives, walnuts, almonds, and soybean oil are helpful. All fruits, with the exception of strawberries, are also beneficial.

When there is not enough acid in the stomach it creates a condition where digestion is hindered. This is often caused by overworking the stomach glands until they go on strike and do not produce enough acid necessary for digestion. Liquids are helpful for this condition, but not at meal time, as the gastric juice is already to weak to work properly. Although, two ounces of lemon juice or six ounces of grapefruit or pineapple juice taken at meals, will help supplement the hydrochloric acid in the stomach and aid in digestion.

The following list contains things that contribute to indigestion.

1) Eating too fast
2) Overeating
3) Meals too close together
4) Eating between meals
5) Eating late at night
6) Eating when tired, nervous or depressed
7) Condiments
8) Soft drinks, tea, coffee, cocoa
9) Fresh yeast bread
10) Vinegar—1 teaspoon stops digestion of starch, hinders digestion of protein
11) Fried foods
12) Combining fruits and sugar
13) Combining fruits and vegetables
14) Drinking at meals or too much liquid foods

The stomach is a very delicate organ as are all the organs involved in digestion. Care should be taken to insure that these organs will properly perform their specific functions. This in turn will insure that the food we eat will be digested and absorbed properly to fill the needs that the body has.

Next we will follow the food as it travels from the stomach into the small intestine where most of the digestion and absorption takes place.

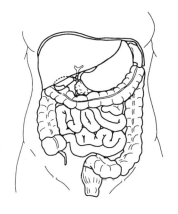

THE SMALL INTESTINE

Small intestine

To continue the study of the digestive system, we will follow the food as it leaves the stomach and enters the small intestine. The small intestine is about 21 to 22 feet long in an average adult. It coils and folds around so that it fits compactly into the lower abdomen. The first section of the small intestine, about a foot long and C-shaped, is called the duodenum. The middle section is called the jejunum, and the last section is the ileum.

The pylorus, a sphincter muscle

Between the stomach and the duodenum is a sphincter muscle called the pylorus. This is a Greek word which when translated into English means simply gate keeper. The pylorus inspects the food being digested in the stomach and at proper intervals allows food that has been prepared, to pass into the small intestine for complete digestion. When the stomach is empty this gate remains open. Water and other liquids at or near the temperature of the body will pass quickly into the intestine.

When the digestive process is started by chewing food, the gastric juices are released into the stomach. These juices coming in contact with the pylorus cause it to contract and close. This gate must be closed and remain closed to retain the food in the stomach until it is digested enough to be sent into the small intestine. Only when the gastric juices in the stomach which are acidic have been neutralized by the alkaline bile and pancreatic juice will the pylorus relax to let food through. Through this method, only small amounts of food are allowed into the intestine at a time. This is where the complete and finished work of digestion takes place.

Problems with unbalanced acidity

In the last lesson we studied the problems that occur in the stomach when there is too much or too little acid. This also affects the pylorus and causes trouble in the small intestine. If there is too much acid the pylorus contracts so tight that food is not passed through to the duodenum. This retention of food in the stomach aggravates the gastric glands so they secrete more acid. This will then cause the movement of the stomach muscles to become so violent that the acid is forced through the esophagus to the mouth. In the event of not enough gastric juice in the stomach, the pylorus remains open and the food moves through the stomach before the necessary digestion takes place. This, in turn, causes digestion in the intestine to be hindered. Often, when this is the case, a bowel movement occurs within 30 minutes of eating, discharging food that was just eaten.

Digestive juices

Both the liver and the pancreas secrete digestive juices into the duodenum through the bile duct. The pancreas pours one to two pints of juice into the duodenum daily. The liver produces a thick green fluid called the bile which aids in digesting fats by causing them to digest in water. We will study the liver, pancreas, and gall-bladder more completely in a later lesson. The duodenum passes the food along to the rest of the intestine. The last two sections of the small intestine have millions of glands in the walls that excrete an additional five pints of digestive juices a day to aid in digestion.

Villi

The walls of the small intestine are lined with an estimated five million villi. The villi, small finger-like projections, absorb the nutrients from the soupy mixture in the intestine that are then sent through the blood stream to the entire body. Within each villus is a network of capillaries. Amino acids and simple sugars pass through the walls of the villi into these capillaries. There are also lymph vessels in each villus which absorb the fat nutrients. It is important that these villi are kept in working condition to allow the absorption of nutrients that the body needs. They can become clogged by too much concentrated protein. Also, mineral oil cannot be absorbed because it is a lubricant and coats the villi so they cannot absorb food into the blood. These villi are so small that one of them can absorb only an ounce of liquid in sixty years. Altogether when functioning properly they absorb about six quarts of liquid daily.

Cellulose

When the nutrients are absorbed into the villi, all that remains is cellulose which the human body is unable to digest. Cellulose passes from the small intestine to the large intestine or colon where it is combined with waste material deposited in the large intestine by the blood and then removed from the body. We will continue the study of the digestive system in the next lesson.

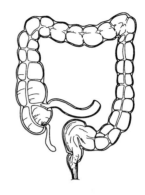

THE LARGE INTESTINE

So far in the study of the digestive system we have learned how the mouth, stomach, and the small intestine all do their part in the digestion of the food. In this lesson we learn about the large intestine or colon, the last organ in the digestive system. The condition of the colon has much to do with good health, in fact more than most people would ever imagine. This will be shown more as we learn about the colon.

Large intestine

The colon is not as long as the small intestine. It is only about four to six feet in length and two inches in diameter. There are three parts to the colon; the ascending colon, the transverse colon, and the descending colon. Also, at the bottom of the descending colon is a section called the pelvic colon. The ascending colon extends from the lower right abdomen to the liver. The transverse section passes across the abdomen from the liver on the right to the spleen on the left. The descending portion of the colon descends from the spleen and left hip bone to the pelvic colon which connects with the rectum.

Location and size

Just as the pylorus holds the food in the stomach until it is ready for the duodenum, the ileocecal sphincter holds the food in the small intestine until digestion is completed and the absorption of nutrients takes place. The amount of food eaten daily that is water-free and digestible weighs about a pound and a half. Only a small amount of this food is usually found in the material that is passed to the colon. Most of the matter passed into the colon is cellulose, the fibrous carbohydrate in plant foods. Also, a considerable amount of water (90%), and mucus with certain substances excreted by the liver in the bile, pass to the colon.

Purpose

The function of the first half of the colon is to reduce the amount of matter by absorbing a part of the water and needed chemicals. This reduces the amount of material in the colon by more than half. The function of the last half of the colon is to transmit and dispose of the waste from the body. Not only does the colon get rid of the waste from the digestive system, but the blood deposits excretory waste matter into the colon. The colon must dispose of this also.

Emptying of the colon every twenty-four hours

Because the colon has so much waste in it, it should, under normal conditions, discharge its contents at least three times a day or once for each meal eaten. When all parts of the alimentary canal are functioning properly this would occur in the following manner. Breakfast should leave the stomach and reach the lower part of the small intestine in four to five hours. When dinner is eaten, the vigorous action of the alimentary canal pushes the breakfast into the middle part of the colon. This should be accomplished in nine to ten hours from breakfast. Before supper the breakfast residue slowly works its way to the lower end of the colon. The vigorous peristaltic waves put in motion by supper sweep the dinner residue into the colon and passes the breakfast residue to the lower colon to be eliminated. The stimulus from awaking and rising often produces a bowel movement before breakfast when the dinner residue is discarded. Again, the action of the peristaltic waves from eating breakfast discharge the supper residue. Thus in twenty-four hours the colon has been swept clean of all the body wastes and food residue.

Putrification

When the colon is thus kept clean there is no time for any putrification to take place. If the colon is not kept clean in this way the body waste and food residue that is kept in the colon over twenty-four hours putrifies and the blood then absorbs this pollution into the system. The liver, lungs, kidneys and skin must then try to eliminate this waste which the colon failed to dispose of. This places an extra burden on these organs which not only overworks them to the point of wearing out, but also greatly hinders the functions they are to perform.

Results of meat in the diet

It is especially unhealthy when the colon is not emptied after every meal that is eaten when meat is a part of the diet. The colon is loaded with undigested remnants of flesh which under go the same changes which occur in the decaying carcass of a dead animal when left to itself. In this way the system is flooded with poisons which result in disease and death.

The normal amount of time it takes for the food to travel through the digestive system from when it first enters the alimentary canal until it enters the colon is approximately eight hours. This is a distance of nearly twenty-five feet. It stands to reason that the food residue should move the last five feet, only one-fifth as far, in at least one-half the time or four hours. Why should the food residue remain in the colon for forty or more hours, considering that the colon's function is to eliminate this waste and that the absorption of nutrients was completed in the small intestine? This unnecessary delay creates the opportunity for putrefactive poisons to develop and these poisons are the prime factors in the development of chronic disease.

The time that is required for the food to travel from the start of the digestive system until elimination is called transit time. Any transit time that is longer than twenty-four hours is constipation. The average transit time in America is 72 hours, in Australia it is 41 hours and in Africa it is 36 hours. The transit time is directly related to the percentage of chronic disease in a country.

The following list of complaints occur from occasional constipation:

General

Coated tongue	Migraine
Foul breathe	Asthma
Indigestion	Gallstones
Dizziness	Arthritis
Constant fatigue	Diabetes
Loss of pep	Colitis
Muddy complexion	Hemorrhoids
Acne	High blood
Insomnia	pressure
Nervousness	Lowered resistance
Absent-mindedness	Premature old age
Inability to	Pernicious anemia
concentrate	by weakening
Mental depression	gastric glands
Epilepsy	Cancer
Headache	

21

This seems enough, but after a few years of constipation the following occurs:

Group two

Infections in these organs:

Colon	Bladder
Appendix	Tonsils
Small Intestine	Teeth
Pancreas	Gums
Stomach	Sinuses
Gallbladder	Mastoids
Arteries	Lungs
Kidneys	(Tuberculosis)
Liver	

You may think this is the last of it, but the worst is yet to come. After living in this manner for years, degenerative changes appear, such as:

Group three

Degenerative changes in:

Thyroid glands	Gums
Adrenal glands	Teeth
Heart	Uterus
Kidneys	Ovaries
Liver	Breasts
Pancreas	Testes
Ductless glands	Prostate
Nerves	Arteries
Eyes	Lymphatic tissue
Ears	of nasopharynx
Skin	Blood-making organs
Fat	Spinal cord
Hair	accompanying anemia

Ways to avoid constipation

By now I am sure you want to know what causes constipation and how it can be avoided. There are three main causes of constipation:

1) Wrong habits, which include failure to heed promptly the call of nature, lack of exercise, poor posture, and a sour stomach or indigestion.

2) Elements are left out of food which would cause action in the muscles of the colon. The elements that are essential are cellulose, minerals, and vitamins with enough water.

3) Elements which hinder proper elimination include the following thirteen points:

a) Refined grains, chief of which is white flour and all foods of which it is an ingredient; polished rice and all other refined cereal foods; corn starch.

b) Faulty methods of cooking vegetables.

c) Meat, fish and fowl, eggs.

d) Dairy milk.

e) Chocolate, cocoa, tea, coffee.

f) Drinking with meals.

g) Cheese, "ripened" cheeses are the worst kinds.

h) Indigestion.

i) Fried foods.

j) Highly seasoned foods.

k) Pepper, mustard, horseradish, and all irritating condiments.

l) Tobacco, alcohol, opium, sleep-producing drugs.

m) Hasty eating.

Now the laxative program that all should follow for the colon to function properly includes:

Laxative program

1) Use whole grain flours and cereals which are rich in cellulose, minerals, and vitamins.

2) Cook all vegetables without loss of minerals and vitamins.

3) Eat freely of vegetables, especially the coarse, leafy ones.

4) Get a liberal order of raw vegetables daily.

5) Eat freely of fruit. Most fruits are more or less laxative.

6) Use soy bean milk in place of cow's milk.

7) Use soy bean or other imitation cheese in place of dairy cheese.

8) Have meals at regular hours and take time to eat them.

9) When it is possible to do so, dinner should be eaten at noon and a very light meal eaten at night.

10) Ripe olives are very helpful, and can be eaten at every meal with much benefit.

11) Using zwieback is better than using regular bread.

12) Drink water early in the morning to maintain regularity.

Some foods that are especially helpful in relieving constipation are: prunes, pears, figs, apricots, all cooked greens, raw cabbage, raw celery, prune juice, grape juice and fresh apple juice. Also, exercise, such as a walk after each meal is beneficial.

Now we can understand just how important it is to keep the colon functioning properly at all times. To sum this up a quote from Dr. Jamieson, of New York, is appropriate, "If we would keep the stomach and bowels clean we would avoid every ill known except those due to accident." *Abundant Health*, p. 121.

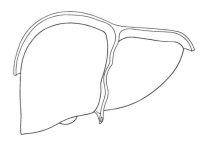

THE LIVER

The liver is one of the busiest organs in the body. It is the largest internal organ and it is also a gland, which also makes it the largest gland in the body. It is a marvelous mechanism, a whole laboratory in itself.	**The Liver**
The liver is located directly under the diaphragm with the majority on the right side of the abdomen and extends past the center to the left side. It is protected by the ribs in front and back. In an adult the liver weighs three to four pounds and is dark red or chocolate colored. The liver is divided into four lobes, or sections, with the two principal sections on the underside. The right section is much larger than the left.	
There are so many functions of the liver that it is quite complex. It is a vital organ and death will occur in eight to twenty-four hours after the liver stops functioning.	**Purpose**
One of the important functions of the liver is to manufacture bile which aids in the digestion that takes place in the small intestine. One pint or more of bile is excreted into the small intestine daily. Bile is secreted by the liver constantly and some of this is stored in the gall bladder. When digestion is taking place the bile is released into the intestine through a tube called the common bile duct. Bile helps the digestive juice remain alkaline. It also aids the pancreatic juice in digesting fats. When the liver does not excrete bile a condition called jaundice occurs. The skin and other tissues turn yellow and food cannot be completely digested.	**Produces bile**
Blood is received in the liver from the stomach and intestines through the portal vein. When this blood passes through the capil-	

laries of the liver it is freed of waste and poisons. The liver also removes from the blood carbohydrates in the form of simple sugar, and changes it into glycogen. Glycogen is stored in the liver, muscles, and skin. It can promptly be converted into glucose when energy is needed by other organs. This is especially essential for the brain, which cannot store glucose and depends upon the liver for a steady supply.

Responds to insulin

The hormone insulin, poured into the blood by the pancreas, tells the liver when to remove the excess sugar from the blood and turn it into glycogen. In this way the liver glycogen regulates the level of sugar in the blood. Diabetes results from the inability to produce insulin and\or the liver not being able to react to the insulin. Resulting in an excessive amount of glucose in the blood.

The liver also stores vitamins A, D, and those of the Bcomplex group, plus minerals. The liver itself contains B_{12} which is necessary for the normal production of the red blood cells. These vitamins and minerals are released from the liver when the body needs them elsewhere in the system.

Helps the blood

There are three main blood proteins that the liver makes. Albumin decreases the flow of blood through the walls of the capillaries. It also helps prevent edema, which is an excess of fluid in the cells. Globulin contains immune bodies that provide the body with a resistance to disease. And fibrinogen is the substance that causes the blood to clot.

Forms urea

Another important function of the liver is to form urea from a nitrogen substance which is derived from protein foods. When the protein is digested in the stomach the blood carries the nitrogen substances to the liver. After the urea is formed in the liver, the liver then releases it into the blood were it is delivered to the kidneys. The urea is then excreted from the body through the urine. It is plain to see how an intake of too much protein is a burden on the liver and kidneys. Urea is a waste matter and too much of this will clog the system and poison it.

Ways to harm the liver

The following a is a list of ways that we can cause harm to the liver or hinder it from performing its functions properly.

1) Lack of air. "Stomach, liver, lungs, and brain are suffering for want of deep, full inspirations of air." —*2 Testimonies*, p. 67.

2) Overeating. "They closely apply their minds to books, and eat the allowance of laboring men....The liver becomes burdened, and unable to throw off the impurities of the blood, and sickness is the result." —*3 Testimonies*, p. 490.

3) Clothing that is too tight. "Woman's dress should be arranged so loosely upon the person, about the waist, that she can breathe without the least obstruction...The compression of the waist weakens the muscles of the respiratory organs...The heart, liver, lungs, spleen, and stomach are crowded into a small compass, not allowing room for the healthful action of these organs." —*Healthful Living*, p. 122.

4) A lack of exercise. "The studied habit of shunning the air and avoiding exercise, closes the pores, —the little mouths through which the body breathes,—making it impossible to throw off impurities through that channel. The burden of labor is thrown upon the lungs, kidneys, etc., and these internal organs are compelled to do the work of the skin." —*2 Testimonies*, p. 524.

5) The use of drugs. "The disease which the drug was given to cure may disappear, but only to reappear in a new form, such as skin diseases, ulcers, painful, diseased joints, and sometimes in a more dangerous and deadly form. The liver, heart, and brain are frequently affected by drugs, and often all these organs are burdened with disease....These organs, which should be in healthy condition, are enfeebled, and the blood becomes impure." —*Healthful Living*, p. 185, 186.

Now that we have looked at some of the things that are harmful to the liver, let us look at ways we can improve the functioning of the liver and help it to do the work it must do for a healthy system.

Ways to aid the liver

1) Exercise in the fresh air. "Morning exercise, in walking in the free, invigorating air of heaven, or cultivating flowers, small fruits, and vegetables, is necessary to a healthful circulation of the blood. It is the surest safeguard against colds, coughs, congestions of the brain and lungs, inflammation of the liver,...and a hundred other diseases." —*Healthful Living*, p. 131.

2) Useful employment. "Useful employment would bring into exercise the enfeebled muscles, enliven the stagnate blood in the system, and arouse the torpid liver to perform its work. The circulation of the blood would be equalized, and the entire system invigorated to overcome bad conditions." —*Healthful Living*, p. 134.

3) Bathing. "Bathing helps the bowels, stomach, and liver, giving energy and new life to each." —*3 Testimonies*, p. 70.

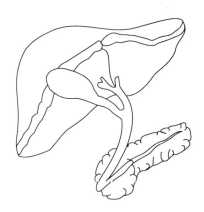

THE GALLBLADDER

Stores bile

The gall bladder is a small pouch that stores bile which is produced by the liver. It is pear shaped and rests on the underside of the right section of the liver. The gall bladder can hold up to one and a half ounces of bile at any one time.

Location

The gall bladder is connected to the liver and duodenum by a series of ducts that form a Y. The hepatic duct comes from the liver to the common bile duct and the cystic duct connects the gall bladder to the common bile duct. The common bile duct enters the pancreatic duct which is connected to the duodenum.

Purpose

Bile is constantly made by the liver. When digestion is in progress, this bile flows from the liver through the hepatic duct to the common bile duct. When digestion is not in progress, bile flows from the liver through the hepatic duct to the cystic duct which enters the gall bladder where the bile is stored. Because of this the gall bladder is necessary as it stores the excessive bile. When bile is not needed in the small intestine a small sphincter muscle, tightens around the opening between the common bile duct and the duodenum stopping the flow of bile into the small intestine. This causes the bile to be forced into the gall bladder where it is stored until, upon endocrine command, it is released into the common bile duct to go to the duodenum. The endocrine command comes in response to the presence of unemulsified fats in the duodenum.

Gallstones

If the bile becomes stagnate or filled with impurities, it will become concentrated and gallstones are formed. Gallstones are made of cholesterol, a kind of alcohol that is in animal fats. Some of the main causes that produce gallstones are: too much sugar, greasy foods, and too much protein. The use of bicarbonate of soda and the lack of water in the system are also contributing factors. Since the liver makes the bile, the liver must be kept in proper health resulting in good bile. Overeating and not drinking enough water overload the liver. Overeating results in the liver being burdened and unable to throw off the impurities of the blood. Not enough water causes the blood to be unable to remove urea, waste from protein, and other wastes from the liver. Therefore these impurities are passed on in the bile and gallstones are formed.

When a stone is formed it may become stuck in the duct and cause great pain in trying to pass to the duodenum. If the stone remains in the duct the flow of bile may be cut off, resulting in jaundice and uncompleted digestion.

Ways to eliminate gallstones

There are several simple things to do to help in the case of gallstones. The diet must be highly alkaline (see alkaline food chart in appendix) to prevent further formation of gallstones. A fruit juice diet of oranges and grapefruit is especially helpful since these juices are cleansing in nature. Hot fomentations over the liver will help relieve the pain.

How important it is that we take care of each organ so that they will all work together and function properly. It is easy to understand how improper eating habits, such as too much food or the wrong kinds of foods, can overload the liver which in turn will cause a negative reaction in the gall bladder. If people would stop eating acid-forming foods and eat alkaline foods, any case of gallstones could be cured.

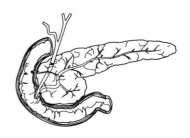

THE PANCREAS

Gland

The pancreas is a gland that is part of the endocrine system. The glands of the endocrine system control many of the body's functions through chemical substances called hormones, which these endocrine glands create. For example the stomach produces a hormone called gastrin which acts on certain cells in the stomach, causing these cells to secrete the necessary acid for digestion.

Location

The pancreas is located in the center of the abdomen behind the stomach and transcending colon. It is also nestled between the kidneys and extends to the spleen on the left side. The duodenum, the first part of the small intestine, loops around the pancreas. The pancreas is six to eight inches long, one and a half inches wide and one inch thick. It is a pinkish-yellow color.

Functions

The pancreas has two functions. One is to produce pancreatic juice which aids in the digestion process. This juice is released into the duodenum through the same duct as the bile. The pancreatic juice contains three enzymes, trypsin, amylase, and lipase. Trypsin breaks down proteins, amylase changes starch into a simple sugar, and lipase splits fats into fatty acids and glycerin. If the six salivary glands are removed from the mouth the pancreatic juice can split the starch in the small intestine. When the gastric juices of the stomach fail to digest the protein the pancreatic juice can do this also. (This creates an extra burden on these organs and is not the ideal way to digest the above mentioned nutrients.)

Produces insulin

The other function of the pancreas is to produce insulin and glucagon. The pancreas is unique in that it is both an endocrine and exocrine gland. Exocrine glands release their secretions into the system through ducts. Endocrine glands do not have ducts through which to release their secretions, but pour their secretions directly into the blood stream which distributes them. The endocrine cells in the pancreas are called alpha cells. They produce a hormone called glucagon. Glucagon causes stored glucose, which is called glycogen, to break down into the blood stream thus raising the level of blood sugar. The exocrine cells in the pancreas are called beta cells. They produce the hormone insulin. Insulin controls the level of blood sugar, enables the body to store and burn sugar properly. Insulin is also needed by the cells to help them use glucose, which is their main fuel. Thus through these processes the level of sugar in the blood is regulated. Four-fifths of the pancreas can be removed without causing an ill effect in the amount of insulin produced that is needed in the body.

Causes of diabetes

When the pancreas does not produce enough insulin, excess sugar accumulates in the blood, this is called diabetes. There are other things that contribute to diabetes besides the lack of insulin, such as an overworked liver. Also, an unbalanced diet, consisting mainly of sugars, fats, and starches also is a cause of diabetes.

An excess of insulin in the body causes hyperinsulinism. This makes the blood sugar level too low, which results in hunger, weakness, excessive perspiration, double vision and eventually a coma.

One reason for diabetes developing, is the system has to much acid and not enough alkaline. Therefore, it is important to eat enough alkaline food, to return the pancreas to health and maintain that health. Some foods especially helpful to diabetes are: all greens, cabbage, onions, sprouted lentils, ripe olives, beets, carrots, celery, soybeans, baked potatoes, almonds and walnuts. All fruits tree-ripened in the sun are excellent, but never sweeten them with sugar. Soda decreases the activity of the pancreatic juices, which are used to digest protein, fats, and carbohydrates and therefore should be eliminated.

When it is understood how the pancreas works, the importance of the counsel given to us in Counsels on Diet and Foods becomes plain. It is much clearer how the system reacts to the eating habits of the individual. If the habits are proper the body can function properly, and if they are not correct neither can the organs in the body do their work correctly.

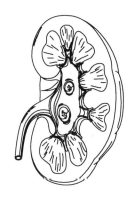

THE KIDNEYS

The kidneys belong to the urinary system, along with the bladder, ureters, and urethra. This system regulates the amount of water in the body and most importantly cleans the blood of wastes.

Part of the urinary system

The kidneys are located on each side of the abdomen just inside the lowest, back rib. The right kidney is slightly lower to make room for the liver. Each kidney is five inches long, two and one-half inches wide, and one and a half inches thick. The kidney resembles a large, purplish-brown bean with the hollow side facing inward.

Location

The kidneys are the magnificent filters of the blood. Blood passes through the kidneys at the rate of a quart a minute or 1,500 quarts every twenty-four hours. In seven minutes they handle an amount of blood equal to all of the blood in the body.

Purpose

The blood enters the kidney through the artery, which in turn divides into a network of blood vessels as a tree trunk divides into many branches. Each of these blood vessels ends in a tuft of capillaries, where the vital exit of waste takes place. These capillaries are entirely surrounded by a capsule called the glomerulus. When the blood reaches the glomerulus capsule, the blood plasma filters through the thin walls of the capillaries into the glomerulus, where the filtering process continues. Each tubule is so small that it can only process a fourth of an ounce of fluid in sixty years. Each glomerulus and tubule make a whole unit, of which there are two to four million in each kidney.

Glomerulus a filtering system

Once in the tubules the fluid is changed to become urine. The water is then returned to the bloodstream, along with the substances important to the body. If there is an excess of these substances; glucose, amino acids, and salts, the excess is allowed to escape into the urine. Therefore the kidneys help to maintain a proper level of each of these substances in the blood stream that the body needs. In twenty-four hours the glomerulus extracts sixty quarts of fluid from the blood, which flows into the tubules. The tubules return all of this to the blood stream except about two quarts which are eliminated into the bladder as urine. In this wonderful way the blood in the body is continually being cleansed of impurities.

Alkaline–acid balance

Also, filtered through the glomeruli, are acids and alkalies. The proper pH of the body is maintained through the kidneys. When the blood becomes to acidic the hydrogen ions move into the tubules and are removed in the urine. If the blood is to alkaline the hydrogen ions are reabsorbed into the blood stream to preserve the proper acid–alkaline balance of the blood.

Necessity of water

There are several things that lead to problems with the kidneys. One of the most important and the easiest to remedy, is furnishing the system with enough water. At least two quarts are needed every day for the kidneys to properly eliminate the body's wastes. Water is necessary for the wastes to be filtered through the walls of the glomerulus so they may be removed in the urine. Without enough water the kidneys are handicapped in the removal of wastes from the blood stream.

When there is not enough water the urine becomes so concentrated that mineral salts are not kept in solution as is required and kidney stones may result.

Effects of poison

Poison is any substance that is harmful to the body or that inhibits the functions of the system. Poison put into the system causes two different problems in the kidneys. The kidney cells were designed to handle only the waste caused by the cells creating energy. When poison is added to the system the kidneys have the extra burden of trying to eliminate the poison as well as the cell waste. The poison also kills kidney cells and then the remaining cells in the kidneys must work harder to do the filtering job. The kidney cells work in shifts—part of them working and a part resting. Therefore when cells in the kidneys are destroyed the remaining cells have less time to rest.

Another problem that occurs is the formation of kidney stones. They are formed by the use of acid-forming foods, white flour products, sugar, meat, tea, coffee, condiments and spices, and vinegar. Overeating is also a main cause of these stones forming. When overeating occurs the liver becomes over burdened and cannot change the excess of digested proteins, carbohydrates, and fats into more usable forms and they are passed to the kidneys. Since these are not broken down into wastes that the kidney was designed to handle they in turn cause inflammation and the formation of kidney stones.

Diuretic drugs act by overtaxing or poisoning the kidneys and thus are especially harmful to the kidneys. The following are four ways that diuretic drugs work:

1) Increasing blood pressure in the kidneys which forces the fluid into the urine collecting ducts. Drugs that do this are those that increase arterial pressure and digitalis types which raise the cardiac output.

2) Interfere with the reabsorption of water or other substances. Mercurial diuretics interfere with sodium and chloride being returned to the blood stream and results in water being retained in the kidney tubules. Thiazide causes more sodium and chloride to be eliminated thus increasing the urine. These types of drugs are toxic.

3) Increase the solid materials in the tubules which requires excess water to remove these solids from the kidneys.

4) Cause the dilation of arterioles within the kidney. Caffeine dilates the arterioles that go to the tiny tubules. This permits an increase in the amount of blood to flow into the tubules thus increasing urine output.

There are two things that place a burden upon the kidneys, according to Ellen White. The use of vinegar and the use of too much liquid foods. The system needs solid food to function properly. The digestive system especially needs fiber to remove the wastes left from digestion.

Things that are helpful to the kidneys are:

1) Exercise, this stimulates the kidneys to work properly.

2) Water, they need this to filter the wastes out of the blood.

3) Fresh air, this will stimulate the kidneys due to the abundance of oxygen in the blood.

4) Alkaline foods, sufficient alkaline foods help in keeping the blood balanced and keeps the kidneys from having too much acid to eliminate.

5) Bathing, stimulates the kidneys and keeps the pores clean and working so that the kidneys do not have to do extra work in eliminated the wastes that are eliminated through the pores of the skin.

6) And making sure one does not eat more food than necessary.

Truly, we can see that the wonderful organism of the kidneys was created by God and is sustained by His power. Let us each be thankful for the wonderful way in which we were made and do our best to keep the body's machinery in working order.

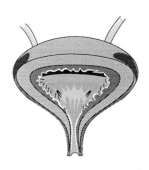

THE BLADDER

In the last lesson we learned how the kidneys filter the urine from the blood and return to the blood the needed substances. Optimum health depends upon regular elimination of the body's waste products. In this study we continue with the urinary system and learn what occurs to the urine once the kidneys have removed it from the blood.

Completion of urinary system

The bladder is located in the lower pelvic cavity near the front. It is an expandable bag, that expands as the urine flows into it. The walls of the bladder contain smooth muscles that are very elastic. As the urine flows into the bladder the walls expand, and when a large amount of urine has stretched the walls enough, nerve endings in the walls are stimulated. When these nerves are stimulated they send messages to the central nervous system of the need to empty the bladder or urinate.

Location and function

When the urine is removed from the blood, in the glomerulus it then flows into the ureters. The ureters are two tubes that stretch from the kidneys in the upper abdomen to the bladder in the lower pelvic cavity allowing the urine to pass from the kidneys to the bladder. Urine constantly flows from the kidneys to the bladder as the kidneys are constantly filtering blood.

Attached to kidneys

At the base of the bladder are two sphincter muscles that stop the release of the urine. These muscles may be relaxed to allow the passing of urine from the bladder into the urethra, which is a tube that leads to the outside of the body. In this manner the system is freed of urine.

Sphincter muscles

Urine is the liquid wastes of the body. Urine is heavier than water and is usually slightly acid. It is made up of water, urea, creatinine,

Contents of urine

uric acid, and inorganic salts. Other things such as sugar, albumin, and blood in the urine indicate a problem else where in the body.

Problems of the bladder

There are several problems that can occur concerning the bladder. One is inflammation of the bladder. When this occurs there is a burning pain in the area of the bladder. Other symptoms can include: frequent urination, the desire to eliminate even when unable to and even when the bladder is empty. There may also be a fever, little or no appetite, and a great thirst. Still other symptoms are that the urine is cloudy, acid, contains mucus and sometimes a red sediment.

Causes

This problem of inflammation is caused by excess acid, which is created by too much starch and sugar in the diet. Also, when waste matter is absorbed by the blood as a result of putrefaction in the colon, inflammation may occur. To reduce the acid, which is causing this inflammation, a fruit diet is the best means of cleansing the system. Fruit is rich in alkaline salts and helps to overcome acidity. The best fruit is grapes as they have the greatest internal cleansing properties, and aid in the elimination of acid from the system, thus aiding the kidneys. Two to three quarts of water need to be taken daily so the urine will not be acid concentrated. The above instructions also apply for scalding or burning urine.

Inability to urinate

The inability to urinate is caused by inflammation and swelling inside the bladder. In severe cases the neck of the gland swells shut causing an obstruction in the exit of urine from the bladder. Pain from the enlargement of the bladder can be so severe the person will break out in a sweat, which has the odor of urine. This must be taken care of with herbs, hot and cold fomentations and a tea injected into the bladder.

There can occur a suppression of urine. This happens when the kidneys do not release the urine into the bladder. If this has occurred over several days severe symptoms such as convulsions and extreme pain in the back and bladder occur. Again this can be relieved with fomentations and certain herb teas.

After having studied the systems of the body it can be seen that strict obedience to the eight laws of health is vital in order to maintain total health. Each system is separate, yet they all affect each other. The health of each and every system depends upon the health of each and every organ. God has been so merciful to us to give us the ways to maintain total health. By His grace may we walk in these ways.

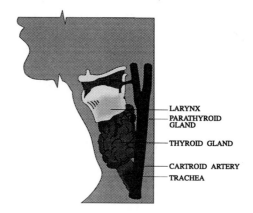

LARYNX
PARATHYROID
GLAND
THYROID GLAND
CARTROID ARTERY
TRACHEA

THE GLANDS

Glands are some of the most important and mysterious parts of the body. Digestion, absorption and utilization of all food elements, and the very existence of the cells depend upon the secretions that the glands send into the body through their various ducts and the blood stream. All mental and physiological activity in the body is possible only because of the functions that the glands perform.

There are two types of glands in the body. The first type are exocrine glands which excrete their secretions into the system through ducts. Included in these are the liver, glands in the stomach, sweat glands, salivary glands, and the pancreas which is also an endocrine gland. (See the section on the pancreas for information concerning its functions.) Since these have already been discussed this lesson will focus on the second type, the endocrine glands. They are referred to as the endocrine system.

The endocrine system is made up of glands that secrete their substances directly into the bloodstream. The endocrine glands produce hormones. Hormones are chemical substances that stimulate and influence the activity of other cells and organs in the body.

The endocrine glands are located throughout the body. A closer look at each gland will tell where they are located and the purpose of each individual gland.

The pituitary gland is often referred to as the master gland. It is located at the center of the skull and hangs from the base of the brain. It is about the size of a cherry. The pituitary gland is not an independent gland. It releases the hormones that are secreted in response to a chemical command from the brain. The pituitary gland

Importance of all glands

Exocrine and endocrine glands

Pituitary gland

receives the chemical command from the hypothalamus. The hypothalamus is located just above the pituitary gland and is responsible for regulating many body functions. It aids in regulating hunger, sleep, thirst, body temperature, sexual drive, and the female menstrual cycle.

Three parts of the pituitary gland

There are three main parts or lobes of the pituitary gland. The front lobe produces many different hormones. Some of these hormones regulate other endocrine glands including the sex glands, thyroid gland, and the adrenal gland. The most important function of the front lobe is the regulation of growth for the whole body. When the front lobe is diseased or removed the body will not develop properly.

The rear lobe stores and releases two hormones. Oxytocin is a hormone that helps in the delivery of a baby and aids in the release of milk from the mammary glands. Vasopressin is an antidiuretic hormone which is necessary to prevent the loss of excess water from the kidney.

The middle lobe produces a hormone, intermedin, which darkens the pigment of the skin.

Thyroid gland

The thyroid glands are located in the front of the neck. It consists of two lobes one on each side of the windpipe. The thyroid gland removes iodine from the blood stream and combines it with other chemicals in the thyroid to make a hormone called thyroxine. Thyroxine is used by the cells in the body to regulate the rate at which the cells use oxygen and nutrients to create energy and heat. Thus body metabolism is maintained. Under the surface of the thyroid gland are four parathyroid glands. These glands produce a hormone that regulates the levels of calcium and phosphorus in the blood stream and the bones.

Adrenal glands

The adrenal glands are located one on top of each kidney. Each adrenal gland consists of two glands, one inside the other. The inner gland, or medulla, which is controlled by the nervous system secretes the hormone adrenalin. When the nervous system reacts to intense emotions, it causes the adrenal gland to pour large amounts of adrenalin into the bloodstream. This adrenalin in turn causes the "fight or flight" reaction throughout the body. In this reaction the heart is stimulated, blood pressure rises, the pupils widen, and blood is shunted to the most vital organs and to the skeletal muscles. The bronchial tubes dilate to allow quicker and greater amounts of breathing. The liver releases more sugar into the bloodstream and the brain burns more oxygen. This provides the excess energy necessary for the emergency. It also causes the muscles of the arteries to contract thus slowing bleeding from wounds.

The outer part of the gland, or cortex, secretes hormones which regulate the metabolism of carbohydrates, proteins, and fats. Some of these hormones also regulate the mineral, salt, and water balance of the body. Cortisone is one of the hormones secreted by the cortex. Cortisone has a marked effect on the formation and use of sugar in the body. It also increases resistance to colds and other stresses the body must deal with.

Thymus gland

The thymus gland made up of spongy tissue is just above the heart in the chest cavity. It influences the activities of lymphocytes in the spleen and the lymph glands. The thymus is large in infants but becomes much smaller as a person matures.

Sex glands

The sex glands have different functions in the male and female, and are sometimes known as the gonads. They contain cells that function in regard to reproduction and produce hormones which affect various body functions. In the male this hormone, testosterone, stimulates the development of the beard and deep male voice. In the female two of these hormones, estrogen and progesterone, make it possible for women to bear children. The third hormone in the female body, relaxin, aids in relaxing the tissues of the birth passages, thus making them wider.

Minerals vital to glandular function

Glands are so complex and are effected by so many different things that it would be very difficult to simply list what is harmful and what is beneficial to them. But, there is one main thing that is vital for all glandular function. All the glands of the body require minerals to produce hormones and to perform their specific jobs. When there is not enough minerals in the diet, the digestive juices receive the supply that is available. This means that the nerves, tissues, teeth and bones will be mineral deficient and that their functions will be greatly hampered. If this state of mineral deficiency is not remedied eventually the glands become affected. This will in turn cause abnormal body conditions that can only result in disease. Because the body obtains minerals through the food that is eaten it is essential that a variety of fresh, raw food be eaten so the body will receive the necessary minerals.

Vitamin A aids all glands in their work

Also vital to many glandular functions is the vitamin A. It effects all of the above mentioned glands as well as the exocrine glands. Some excellent sources of vitamin A are: kale, dandelion greens, chard, green lettuce, collards, broccoli, mustard greens, beet greens, carrots, sweet potatoes, red tomatoes, green peas, green beans, avocados, apricots, prunes, cantaloupes, bananas, ripe olives, and oranges. Because vitamin A is destroyed by boiling or heating when oxidation occurs it is best to eat the above mentioned foods raw, as much as is possible. These fresh foods are also high in minerals necessary for the glandular functions.

Glands are a very complex system of the body and perform many and varied functions. It is necessary to faithfully follow the principles in each of the eight laws of health to maintain healthy glands so they will function properly and regulate the body correctly.

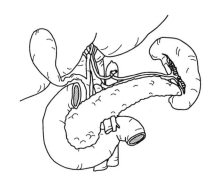

THE SPLEEN

The spleen is classed as a ductless gland. It is part of the circulatory system.

The spleen is the largest of the ductless glands. It lies below the diaphragm, on the left of the stomach and a little behind it. An adult spleen is about 5 inches long and 3 to 4 inches wide, weighing about 7 ounces. The spleen is soft, spongy, and crumbles easily. It is a deep violet-red color.

The spleen has several functions. Red blood cells are stored in the spleen. When the body needs extra blood due to exercise or bleeding the spleen contracts. This contraction sends the stored blood into the blood stream. Red blood cells that are worn out are filtered from the blood stream and broken down by the spleen. Any parts from these worn out red blood cells that are usable the spleen returns to the blood to be used by the bone marrow in production of new red blood cells. If the bone marrow becomes damaged the spleen can function to produce various blood cells. The spleen, along with the bone marrow and liver, continually filter small clots from the blood stream.

Purposes

The spleen produces lymphocytes. Twenty-five percent of the circulating white blood cells are lymphocytes. Lymphocytes are divided into two major classes, B cells and T cells. When a virus enters the body the T cells discover the virus and identify it. The T cells start to multiply and stimulate the production of other T cells and B cells that can fight this particular virus. The T cells also rush to the spleen, where the B cells reside, and signal the B cells to start production of antibodies that will destroy the virus. T cells also signal the immune system to stop when the virus has been de-

Produces lymphocytes

stroyed. Some of the T and B cells that will recall this specific virus, named memory cells, remain in the blood stream to be activated if this particular virus should enter the body again.

The blood enters the spleen through the splenic artery which is very large. The splenic artery divides into six or more branches. These branches continue to be divided into smaller vessels. The smaller vessels empty into the pulp of the spleen. This is where the blood is filtered. After this occurs the blood is collected from the pulp and returned to the blood stream in the same manner it enters the spleen.

Proper blood flow necessary

So many functions depend on the activity of the spleen, especially the immune system. It is necessary for the spleen to function properly so that the body may be in perfect health. In order for the spleen to function properly it must continually receive a good supply of blood. The spleen can receive the needed amount of blood only if the circulation is good. Following the laws of health will ensure a proper circulation of the blood. (See the section on the heart for more information on circulation of the blood.)

Adherence to the ways of God will ensure good health for the entire body including the spleen and its related functions.

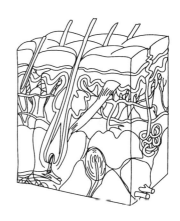

THE SKIN

The skin is the largest organ of the whole body. It belongs to the integumentary system which is made up the skin and its appendages. These appendages include the nails, glands, hair, and breasts.

The skin covers the entire body and in an average adult weighs from 8 to 10 pounds. If the skin of an adult was laid flat it would cover an area of about 22 square feet. A piece of skin the size of a quarter contains a yard of blood vessels, 4 yards of nerves, 25 nerve cells, 100 sweat glands, and more than 3,000,000 cells.

The main purpose of the skin is to provide protection for the body. The skin is a tough, elastic, waterproof covering of the body. The glands in the skin release secretions that prevent the development of bacteria thus protecting the body from infection and disease. The skin also absorbs vitamin D and aids in regulating the temperature of the body.

The skin is made up of two layers. The epidermis which is the top layer and the dermis which is the bottom layer. The dermis is where the functions of the skin occur. The epidermis is made up of several layers of cells. The new skin cells are constantly being formed on the bottom of this layer and then push upward to the surface. As these new cells push upward the old cells on the surface die and flake off. In this manner the skin is constantly being changed or renewed. The epidermis contains melanocytes which are cells that produce a pigment called melanin. The color of the skin depends upon the amount of melanin it contains. The sun stimulates the production of melanin which is why skin exposed to the sun darkens. There are no blood vessels in the epidermis and therefore the cells in this layer of skin receive little nourishment.

Largest organ of the body

Purpose

Two layers of skin

The second layer of skin, called the dermis, lays below the epidermis and is solidly attached to it. This layer of skin contains blood vessels, lymph carrying vessels, hair roots, glands, elastic fiber, different nerve endings and fat.

Oil glands of skin

There are three types of glands located in the dermis. One, the sebaceous glands secrete an oily substance directly into the hair shaft. Each hair of the body is a slender thread-like structure that grows from the bottom of a shaft, or follicle. The cells of hair are modified epidermis cells. The oily substance (sebum) released into the shaft keeps the hair lubricated and not so brittle. Every follicle has a tiny muscle that contracts when stimulated by cold or an emotion such as fear. When this muscle contracts it stands the hair up straight and creates a goose bump. Because sebum is released into the hair shaft only a small amount reaches the outer layer of the epidermis. In this way sebum aids in the lubrication of the outer skin.

Wax glands

The second type of gland is located in the skin of the ear. These glands are called ceruminous glands and excrete a waxy substance. This waxy substance (cerumen) traps foreign materials before they enter the ear.

Sweat glands

The third type of glands that are found in the skin are the sweat glands. Sweat glands (sudoriferous glands) secrete sweat through ducts which lead directly to the surface of the skin. The openings for these ducts are called pores. There are approximately two million sweat glands in the skin of the body. The palms of the hands, soles of the feet, and the armpits contain many large sweat glands. The glands in these areas respond not only when the body is too warm, but also to excitement or nervousness.

Purpose of sweat glands

The sweat secreted is a salty fluid that contains liquid wastes from the system and an antibacterial substance which helps to control the skin flora. Included in the liquid wastes of the sweat are urea, carbon dioxide, and acid. Every day a pint of fluid is removed from the blood by the sweat glands and released through the skin. When it is cool this sweat evaporates as soon as it is formed. This is called insensible perspiration. During hot weather or strenuous exercise the sweat glands will increase production of sweat up to five gallons a day. When this occurs, drops of water accumulate on the skin. This action is called sensible perspiration. The hypothalamus, a part of the brain which has a heat-regulating center, receives impulses from warm blood and from heat receptors in the skin. The hypothalamus in turn sends signals through the nerves to the sweat glands to produce more sweat to release the heat in the body. Since a large percent of sweat is water it is necessary that the body receive sufficient water to be able to remove these impurities through the skin. When there is not enough water received, these wastes must be removed through the other eliminating organs such as the lungs, liver, and kidneys thus placing an additional burden on them and poisoning the system.

Wastes removed through the skin

Once the sweat has evaporated on the skin there is a residue of solid wastes that remain on the skin. These must be removed from the skin by thorough washing so the pores will not become plugged. When the pores are closed they can not breathe or release poison from the system. The poison is then absorbed back into the blood and forced upon the internal organs. The impurities released through the pores are absorbed onto the clothing. The clothing must be cleansed from these impurities or the skin will reabsorb the impurities that have already been secreted. Overeating will clog the entire system including the bloodstream which in turn clogs the skin and its elimination. This will cause eruptions of the skin. A blackhead forms when hard fatty material from the gland blocks the gland's opening.

Dangers of cosmetics

"Many are ignorantly injuring their health and endangering their lives by using cosmetics..When they become heated,....the poison is absorbed by the pores of the skin, and is thrown into the blood. Many lives have been sacrificed by this means alone." *Healthful Living*, p. 189.

Mamma glands

The mamma or breast are present in both the male and female, but usually these glands only develop fully on the female. The mammary glands are modified sweat glands that secrete milk for the newborn instead of sweat. The milk carrying ducts empty into the nipple through which the milk flows to the newborn. The activity and size of the breasts are under the control of a hormone secreted from the endocrine glands.

Nerves of the skin

The skin contains several different types of nerves. These nerves each respond to different sensations of touch, heat, cold, pain, and pressure. The nerves send messages of these sensations to the brain so the brain may monitor the external environment of the body and in turn tell the system to respond as necessary for the well being and comfort of the individual.

Let us determine to keep the skin clean so the body can rid itself of poisons and toxins in a natural way, resulting in cleaner blood and healthier bodies.

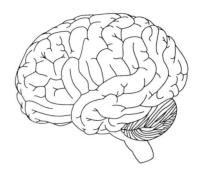

THE BRAIN

The nervous system is the most complicated system of the body. Sensory perception, perception of pain and pleasure, control of the body movements, and the regulation of the body functions all depend upon the nervous system. The nervous system is vital for the development of language, thought, feelings, and memory.

The brain, the spinal cord, and the nerves are all part of this nervous system, which is divided into two parts; the central nervous system and the peripheral nervous system. The brain is the most complex organ of the entire body, and with the spinal cord has ultimate control over the rest of the nervous tissue in the body. The brain and spinal cord are often referred to as the central nervous system because of this control. The peripheral nervous system refers to the nerves throughout the body that collect information and then send it to the central system. The peripheral nervous system then transmits the signal received from the brain and spinal cord to the body.

Nerve cells, called neurons, make up the working parts of the nervous system. The purpose of these neurons is to transmit signals from one part of the body to another. There are three types of neurons, classified according to their functions.

1) Sensory neurons, which convey information from the sense organs to the central nervous system;
2) Integrative neurons, which process the information received from parts of the body;
3) Motor neurons, which initiate voluntary and involuntary actions.

Neurons come in many sizes and shapes, depending upon their functions. The brain neurons are very small, while a neuron cell

Most complicated system

Brain, spinal cord, and nerves

Nerve cells or neurons

running from the lower part of the spinal cord to the toes, may be as long as four feet. Neurons all have the same basic structure. As a cell, neurons have a nucleus which is contained in the round part of the cell called the cell body. A number of fine, root-like fibers, called dendrites, project from the cell body.

How nerve impulses are transmitted

There is a single, long fiber projecting from the cell body called an axon. The axon is the main conducting fiber of a nerve. At the far end of this axon it is divided into a number of branches. Each branch ends in a tiny knob. These knobs are very close to the knobs on a neighboring neuron although they do not touch. This small gap is called a synapse. Messages are transmitted across this gap by chemicals called nerve transmitter substances.

The dendrites, the short fibers, accept the electrical message and send it to the cell body. The cell body then sends the message down the axon where the electrical current jumps across the gap to the dendrites of the neighboring neuron, or to muscles or glands where the message is sent on or that particular command fulfilled.

Some neurons are covered by a thin layer of fatty material called myelin. This is made by special cells that surround the neuron. Myelin covered neurons transmit messages much faster than the uncovered neurons. The covered neurons are capable of transmitting an impulse at the rate of 450 feet per second. Those neurons that are not covered can only transmit an impulse at the speed of three feet per second.

Location of spinal cord

The spinal cord extends from the base of the brain about two thirds of the way down the spinal column. Many nerves branch off from the cord. At the bottom of the cord, nerve fibers continue down within the spinal column. The meninges, which are protective membranes, surround the cord as well as the brain.

Purpose of spinal cord

The spinal cord has two main functions. The first is to act as a two way communication system between the brain and the peripheral system of nerves. The second function of the spinal cord is to control simple reflex actions. When a hand is placed on a hot stove the motor neurons of the spinal cord send signals to the muscles to remove the hand. At the same time other messages travel up to the neck motor nerves and instruct the head to turn toward the pain.

50

While this is happening other signals travel clear to the brain and cause the conscious sensation of heat and pain.

The brain is located in the head. An adult brain weighs approximately 3 pounds. It is surrounded and protected by the bones of the skull, by the meninges, and by the cerebrospinal fluid. The meninges are protective membranes which cover the brain. Four spaces called ventricles, surround the brain and are occupied by the cerebrospinal fluid. The fluid flows from the ventricles through the meninges and back into the blood stream.

Brain

The brain is not a single organ, but has many parts that have different functions, but these parts are all connected. The largest and most complex part of the brain is the cerebrum. The cerebrum composes 85 percent of the brain's weight. There are two hemispheres to the cerebrum that are connected by several bands of nerve fibers called the corpus callosum. Each hemisphere is made up of an outer covering of gray matter, called the cerebral cortex. Under this cerebral cortex is a core of white matter with nerves that connect the cortex to the brain stem, and connect the areas of the cortex together.

Cerebrum composed of two hemispheres

The cerebral cortex starts and stops all voluntary movements of the body. Learning, judgment, creativity and some emotions are the responsibility of the cerebral cortex. The "motor strip" on each hemisphere of the brain is in control of the voluntary movements of the opposite side of the body. Sensations, such as, pain, heat, and cold, are received by the opposite side of the brain. Other areas of the cerebral cortex receive the responses from sight, hearing, taste, and smell.

Cerebral cortex

The left hemisphere of the brain is responsible for producing and understanding speech, reading, writing, and logical thinking. The right hemisphere is involved in creativity, artistic ability, and the emotions.

The brain is also divided in to areas according to location. There is the frontal lobe, located at the top front or directly behind the forehead. This location is where complicated thinking occurs. Mrs. White often refers to this as the intellect, reasoning, or the higher powers. The parietal lobe is located towards the back of the brain. This is where responses to touch and taste occur. The temporal lobe is near the base of the brain and is where the responses from hearing, smell, and vision are transmitted. These last two lobes are referred to in the writings of Mrs. White, as the lower powers or animal passions.

Because the brain through the nervous system controls the vital action of the entire body, it is understood that to have health one must have a properly functioning brain. What are ways that aid in the proper working of the nervous system?

Things that aid the nervous system

The cerebrospinal fluid that flows through the brain is derived from the blood stream. This fluid carries the oxygen and nutrients necessary for the brain cells to create energy to do their jobs and then removes the wastes from these cells.

1) A constant supply of fresh air.

   The brain needs fresh oxygen constantly to remain alive. Brain cells die in five minutes without oxygen. When circulation is cut off to an area of the brain that area dies. This is what happens in a stroke.

2) A constant supply of glucose.

   This glucose is made by the digestive system from the food the body eats. It is necessary to maintain a diet balanced in all nutrients to fulfill this need of the brain.

3) Daily exercise that will increase the circulation.

   Exercise increases the blood flow to the brain thus increasing the oxygen level and decreasing the waste matter so the neurons will function at top capability.

4) Plenty of water.

   The neurons transmit their signals with electrical impulses. These impulses can travel faster when the fluid between the neurons is kept clean and pure with enough water intake.

One of the most important factors that we can control which affects the nervous system is our diet; which includes everything we eat and drink. When the stomach is not properly taken care of there is a direct response on the brain. Notice the following:

When the stomach is:	The brain is:
overloaded	sensitive nerves benumbed, vitality weakened, judgment perverted, thoughts sluggish

given flesh foods	clouded, the intellect inactive, the moral sensibilities blunted
given caffeine	benumbed, injured, irritated, paralysis of mental powers
given milk and sugar together	directly affected due to the entire system being clogged through the blood stream
given food late at night	and nerves are wearied

Another area that can affect the brain is the way that the body is clothed. When the limbs are uncovered and become chilled the blood from the limbs is forced back to the main organs, including the brain. This causes the brain to be congested and inflamed and unable to properly function.

Adherence to all eight laws of health, along with dress reform and every other requirement that God has so bountifully given to us, is essential to return to or maintain perfect health and have a clean, clear, sharp, active mind.

The
8 Laws
of
Health

GOD'S PLAN

G-God's sunshine
O-Open air
D-Daily exercise
S-Simple trust

P-Proper rest
L-Lots of water
A-Always temperate
N-Nutrition

God has given us these laws of health to govern the physical nature and they "are as truly divine in their origin and character as the law of the ten commandments" (*Healthful Living*, p. 21). These laws were given to humanity that "thou mayest prosper and be in health, (3 John 2), but when they are not obeyed disease in some form is the result. "God has formed laws to govern every part of our constitutions, and these laws which He has placed in our being are divine, and FOR EVERY TRANSGRESSION THERE IS A FIXED PENALTY, which sooner or later must be realized." *Healthful Living*, p. 20. God's desire is for the laws of health to be kept, but when they are not followed and disease is the result, He has provided a means to return the body to health. This is a parallel in the physical world of the plan of salvation in spiritual life.

In this series we are going to look at how the eight laws of health give us total health, but even more how they are to be used to restore the body to its best physical condition. In *Ministry of Healing*, p. 127, it states, "EVERY PERSON should have a knowledge of nature's remedial agencies and how to apply them. It is essential both to understand the principles involved in the treatment of the

8 laws of health as Divine as the 10 Commandments

Every person should have this knowledge and a training to properly use it

sick and to have a practical training that will enable one rightly to use this knowledge." We are told in many places that this knowledge is an essential part of education. "It is her (the mother's) right to obtain such a knowledge of the best methods of treating disease that she can care for her children in sickness." *Fundamentals of Education*, p. 75

God's Plan takes time and effort

It is important to remember that God's Plan takes time and effort. "The use of natural remedies requires an amount of care and effort that many are not willing to give. Nature's process of healing and up building is gradual, and to the impatient it seems slow." *Ministry of Healing*, p. 127

Only ONE way of healing that heaven approves of

"There are many ways of practicing the healing art; but there is only one way that Heaven approves. God's remedies are the simple agencies of nature, that will not tax or debilitate the system through their powerful properties." *Healthful Living*, p. 225. This tells us that all around us are different healing methods, but we must live "by every word that proceedeth out of the mouth of God." *Matthew 4:4*. It is necessary for us to use caution and discernment when looking at a method of healing to be sure that we are not deceived by Satan into using a plan or method that is not approved of by God. May God help us as we endeavor to learn and use God's Plan properly.

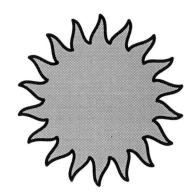

GOD'S SUNSHINE

The sun is a most essential element of life on our planet; it is a mediator of all life on earth. No life can exist or function without sunlight.

Most essential element

What is the sun? Not only does the sun produce light it also is the source of ninety-eight percent of the energy on earth. The way the sun produces energy is that 600 million tons of hydrogen are fused to helium every second and about 4 million tons of hydrogen are converted into energy every second. This produces heat which radiates to the earth through sunlight. Sunlight arrives at the earth approximately 8 minutes after it leaves the sun.

Sun source of energy

This sunlight causes many reactions on earth necessary for life. The air and ocean currents, which air condition the planet, are activated by the sunlight. Water is evaporated from the oceans and returns to the clouds to then water the earth that animal and plant life may live.

Most important, sunlight is the force which nourishes and energizes your body. The environment necessary for our existence is sustained by sunlight. It creates oxygen and carbon dioxide. The temperature and humidity at life-supporting levels are regulated by sunlight.

Energizes the body

The food we eat is developed by sunlight. The plant receives minerals and water through its roots and air through its leaves. With these and chlorophyll, the sun changes the water and carbon dioxide into sugar and invisible oxygen. From the sugar, the plant makes all the nutrients it needs. In this reshuffling the atoms that make up sugar are combined with minerals and supply starch, oil,

Aids in creating plant nutrition

protein, vitamins, and all that is needed in human nutrition. Thus through the plant family the sunlight provides for humans the nutrients necessary for the body to properly function.

Vitamin D

Vitamin D is a nutrient that the sunlight gives directly to the human body. The body has fat in the skin that contains ergosterol, which absorbs ultraviolet rays and changes them to vitamin D. This vitamin is essential because it prevents excretion of calcium and phosphorus, from the intestine. Calcium and phosphorus are needed in the system for healthy teeth and bone development and maitainance. A lack of vitamin D causing low levels of calcium and phosphorus can result in a condition of soft teeth and bones, a weak heart, abnormal metabolism, slow healing of wounds, and the nerves suffer. Vitamin D also aids in the absorption into the body of calcium and phosphorus from the food and regulates the blood levels of these minerals.

Circulatory system benefitted

All of the body systems improve in their functions due to the body receiving sufficient sunlight. The circulatory system is one that receives many benefits. Sunlight increases the circulation and enables the red blood cells to carry more oxygen. There is an increase in cardiac output which lowers the resting heart rate and causes the heart to return to a normal heart beat after exercise much quicker than if no sun is received at all.

Electrifies brain

The nervous system sends commands and messages from the brain throughout the body and sends information collected from the body to the brain. This is done by the nerves sending electrical signals. Since sunlight has an electrifying influence it imparts a healthy tone to the mind and nervous system. The sun also prevents and counteracts mental depression. Since the nerves of the brain control the vital action of every part of the body it is mandatory that they be in proper working condition for the body functions to perform correctly. The nerves are soothed by sunlight and having calm nerves is necessary in order for the nervous system to function properly.

Increases white blood cells

The immune system benefits largely from the sun. One benefit from the sun to the immune system is that the number of white blood cells are increased when the body is in the sunlight. White blood cells do many things to fight infection in the body. Some of them identify the germs, some kill the cells of the body that have been invaded and others stimulate the production of different white blood cells that fight the infection.

One of the specialized white blood cells is gamma globulin. Gamma globulin is one of several proteins in the blood plasma. When an infection begins, the body and the white blood cells manufacture antibodies to fight the infection. Antibodies are mainly composed of gamma globulin. The body is less resistant to disease when the amount of gamma globulin is decreased.

Liver stimulated

The liver, a gland, provides many important functions for the body. It manufactures bile which aids with digestion. Waste and poisons are removed from the blood which pass through the liver. The brain is dependent upon the liver for glucose, which is the fuel for cell energy, since the brain cannot store glucose for itself. Also, the liver stores vitamins A, D, B complex, and some minerals until they are needed else where in the body. By receiving sufficient sunlight the liver is stimulated to properly perform these and other necessary functions and thus the body is benefitted in many ways.

Body functions stimulated

When the pineal gland (a small gland in the brain) receives sunlight through the eyes it in turn benefits the pituitary gland. The pituitary gland controls the hormone production of other endocrine glands including the liver, pancreas, thyroid, and adrenal glands. Thus in allowing sunlight to enter the eye many of the body functions are stimulated.

Natural insulin

The sunlight affects the carbohydrate metabolism in the body as does insulin—sunlight lowers the level of blood sugar in the blood stream when it is to high and raises the level if it is low. This is done in the exact proportion that is needed to maintain the proper level of sugar in the blood stream.

Benefits increased when combined with exercise

It is of interest that many of these beneficial effects of sunlight are increased when a person combines sunbathing with a regular program of physical exercise. For example, fatigue and exhaustion tend to be lessened and the capacity for work is increased. It is now known that part of this is due to an increase of glycogen content in the blood and muscles following exercise in the sunlight.

Increased blood output

The strength of the heart is deepened and steadied when exercise is combined with sunlight. The pulse rate is lowered, because the heart muscle is pumping more blood at each beat. This enables your heart to rest more between beats. And yet, the blood output is increased by an average of 39% for several days after a sunbath.

Blood pressure lowered

A high level of triglycerides, the amount of fats in the blood, and high blood pressure are both lowered by adequate sunlight. Simply taking sunlight on the body will lower the blood pressure by an average of 8%. When a person combines exercise with receiving sunlight high blood pressure is lowered by 15%.

Sunlight and nutrition are intimately connected. What a person eats has a direct effect on how the body reacts to sunlight. A diet of sufficient vitamin A, fresh fruits, vegetables, with the elimination of free fats (grease, oil, etc), greatly lowers the risk of skin cancer from the sun.

Proper sunbathing

Another factor in lowering skin cancer is sunbathing in a proper manner. One should be exposed to the sun only a few minutes at first and then progressively increase the time exposed each day by five to ten minutes until a total of thirty minutes for each side of the body, front and back, is reached. It is important to remember that by exposing a six inch square of the face or hands to an hour of sunlight a day the body receives all the necessary benefits from the sun.

Kills germs

Sunlight benefits both the elderly and the child. The elderly have an increased need of sun because they have less vitality with which to resist unhealthful influences. Since it is known that direct sunlight kills most disease germs in a few minutes, it gives to the elderly an advantage in resisting unhealthful influences besides its other benefits. White blood cells are increased by the sun, thus giving extra help to the system in fighting infections.

The growing child needs sunshine because of the effect it has on their body of creating vitamin D, needed for their developing bones. Sunlight also gives them a healthy glow by increasing their circulation of blood.

Some of the miscellaneous ways that the sun benefits the body are:

1) it promotes the healing of wounds

2) lessens stress by working both through sensory receptors in the skin as well as through psychological factors.

3) kills some germs on exposure.

Just as plants reach to the sun so should we as humans place ourselves in the sun to receive its life-giving, health-dealing power. Sunlight is one of nature's most healing agents. God provides for us the sunlight to keep us healthy and aid in the restoration of health to us all.

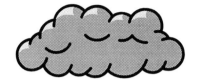

OPEN AIR

Air is the most essential element needed to sustain life. "The strength of the system is, in a great degree, dependent upon the amount of pure, fresh air breathed." *Healthful Living*, p. 171. How can oxygen, which is vital for life, help us to regain and retain our health?

Essential to life

The body is made up of cells. Cells in turn make up tissues and tissues in turn make up the organs of the body. Every function carried on by the body is directly related to the life of the cells. Cells need four things to live and function properly. These essentials are:

Cells require 4 things

1) oxygen—without oxygen the cells die in 3 minutes.

2) water—without water the cells die in a few days.

3) nutrition—without nutrients they die in a few weeks.

4) cleansed—their own wastes must be removed promptly or death will result in a matter of minutes or at the most hours.

Oxygen is one chemical essential for the cells to create energy. This chemical reaction necessary to create energy leaves a carbon dioxide waste residue in the cell. This waste must be removed to ensure healthy cells.

Specialized blood cells carry the oxygen, nutrients, and wastes to and from the different organs of the body to keep them functioning properly. When the lungs fill with oxygen the oxygen molecules seep through the walls of the alveoli, tiny air sacs in the lungs, and enter the blood stream. There the oxygen is connected to the outside of the red blood cells which deliver it to every part of the system. It is then assimilated into the capillaries of the tissues and then into the individual cells. The carbon dioxide is then picked up by the red blood cells and taken back to the lungs where it is eliminated from the system. Since the oxygen is carried on the outside

Oxygen transported on outside of red blood cells

of the red blood cells it is important to keep the blood from being sticky (clumping together of the red blood cells caused by a high fat diet) or the veins and arteries from being clogged. If this happens the oxygen cells are no longer able to ride with the red blood cells and an oxygen deficiency results. The importance of oxygen, healthy blood and proper circulation is realized when it is understood that in virtually every disease there is a low level of oxygen in the cells.

Amount of oxygen in system

Every minute five quarts of blood pass through the lungs receiving fresh oxygen and eliminating the carbon dioxide. This diffusion of oxygen and carbon dioxide from the lungs to the blood requires from one pint to one quart of water daily. Thirty quarts of carbon dioxide are discharged through the lungs every hour. Normally the body contains a little more than one quart of oxygen at any given time. An adult inhales approximately sixteen to eighteen times a minute. In each of these inhalations about one pint of air is received into the lungs.

Negative charged ions in air healthier

The air in our atmosphere is ionized. There are negatively charged oxygen molecules and positively charged carbon dioxide molecules. The more negative charged ions in the air the healthier it is. The outdoor air is negatively charged from the natural ionizing effect of radioactive particles in the atmosphere and the earth's crust. This ionization also occurs from sunshine and the breakup of water droplets by the ocean or near waterfalls. Negative ions are rapidly lost indoors by adhering to walls, air conditioning ducts, and fabric materials. Also, wood burning stoves destroy the negative ions. Therefore to obtain enough oxygen from the air it is necessary to have a continuous supply of fresh air that is negatively charged.

Benefits received from open air

The benefits that are received from having a constant supply of pure, fresh air are:

1) Fresh air purifies the blood, imparts to it a bright color, and sends the blood, a life giving current, to every part of the body.

2) Air soothes the nerves, stimulates appetite, helps digestion, and induces sound, refreshing sleep.

3) Oxygen electrifies the whole system, causes the body to be strong and healthy, and will refresh the system.

4) Air invigorates the vital organs and aids the system in getting rid of an accumulation of impurities.

5) Pure air brings life to the skin as for a lack of air the skin nearly dies.

6) But most important air has a decided influence on the mind, imparting a degree of composure and serenity.

7) Some specific problems that are greatly benefitted by having an abundance of fresh air are: fevers, colds, and lung diseases.

One of the best ways to receive the benefits from fresh air is to go out of doors into the open air and exercise by walking or gardening. This enables the lungs to expand and be filled with the negatively charged oxygen molecules. "Exercise in the open air should be prescribed as a life-giving necessity. And for such exercises there is nothing better than the cultivation of the soil." *Medical Ministry*, p. 233. The amount of oxygen taken in by each breath increases by three times the normal amount when walking.

Walking excellent way to obtain air

Fresh air outdoors is essential to health, but just as important if not more so, is the necessity of a constant supply of pure air indoors. Since the lungs not only expel carbon dioxide but also other waste matter, if this indoor air is not replaced by negatively charged oxygen, it becomes poisonous and causes, among other things, sore throats, lung diseases and liver complaints. This is especially true at night when sleeping in a closed room. Unless there is a supply of fresh air a person will awake unrested and irritable.

Fresh oxygen indoors essential

It is necessary to breathe properly in order for the lungs to be filled with enough fresh oxygen to function properly. When breathing correctly the lungs expand and the diaphragm pushes down into the abdomen. This in turn causes the lower abdomen to extend outward. It is simple to check and see if the breathing is proper. Stand erect yet relaxed and take a breath. Does the lower abdomen extend as the lungs are filled and then return as the air is expelled? It maybe necessary to practice this correct way of breathing until it becomes a natural habit.

Pure, open air is so available and free, and it works wonders for the health of the body. Let us put as much fresh air as possible in our system so we may reap the healthful benefits that God has placed in the atmosphere surrounding us.

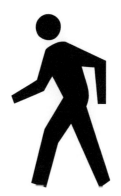

DAILY EXERCISE

The human body may be compared to a well adjusted machine which must have care in order for it to run well. In the last two lessons the benefits from sunshine and open air were reviewed. Exercise in the sunshine and open air is a necessary ingredient for the body to maintain health as well as return to optimum health.

The body is made up of cells. Cells in turn make up tissues and tissues in turn make up the organs of the body. Every function carried on by the body is directly related to the life of the cells. Each muscle in the body is made up of individual muscle cells. Since all cells require energy to function, any movement by these muscle cells requires energy. All cells use amino acids and fatty acids combined with a glucose and oxygen to make energy. Amino acids come from protein and fatty acids come from fats while glucose comes from sugar and oxygen from the air we breathe. Thus for the muscle cells to function they need a sufficient amount of acids, glucose and oxygen. The more energy the muscle cells burn due to exercise the more acids, glucose, and oxygen is needed to allow the cells to continue moving in exercise.

Cells require oxygen to create energy

Oxygen can only be supplied to the muscles through the red blood cells. When muscles are being used in exercise, the heart must pump more blood through the body to supply the need for extra oxygen. This in turn, causes the lungs to be expanded to fill the need of oxygen required by the red blood cells. Therefore increased heart rate and rapid breathing are the result of proper exercise.

Leviticus 17:11 says, "The life of the flesh is in the blood." What is in the blood constitutes life. If there is life in the blood, but bad circulation, the entire system cannot receive the life it needs. Each cell in the body requires nourishment from nutrients and cleansing from its own

Circulation cleanses and supplies nutrition

wastes, to be healthy. Nutrients are delivered to each cell through the blood stream and in turn the wastes are picked up by the blood and deposited in the eliminating organs. Thus we can understand the statement, "Perfect health depends upon perfect circulation." *2 Testimonies*, p. 531. "The more active the circulation the more free from obstructions and impurities will be the blood." *Healthful Living*, p. 178.

How exercise increases circulation

Due to the fact that the muscles are requiring more oxygen to create energy the body naturally increases the amount of oxygen inhaled. The heart rate increases as it pumps the blood, which moves faster now, through the system to supply the necessary oxygen to each muscle. Thus the circulation of the blood is greatly increased. This increase in circulation has a two fold benefit to the body. First, an abundant supply of oxygen is taken not only to the muscles, but to every part of the system. And second, the blood is circulated through the eliminating organs at a much greater amount, thus resulting in an increase in the elimination of the body's wastes. Both of these are essential for good health and healing.

Benefits to heart and lungs

Exercise benefits the whole system, but let us notice in what ways the heart and lungs are especially benefitted from daily exercise. This type of exercise is called cardiopulmonary exercise. (What is involved in cardiopulmonary exercise will be shown later.)

1) It increases the stroke volume, the amount of blood pumped with each heart beat.

2) It decreases the pulse rate, thereby giving the heart more time to rest between beats.

3) It decreases one's risk of death in the event of a heart attack.

4) The lungs are expanded and thus strengthened to supply fresh oxygen to the entire system.

Benefits received due to increased circulation

Perhaps the most important benefit is that of increased circulation. Other benefits realized by the whole body due to the increase of circulation are:

1) The liver, kidneys, and lungs will be strengthened to perform their work.

2) Exercise invigorates the mind.

3) Digestion is aided, a diseased stomach is relieved, and the bowels are strengthened for correct elimination.

4) Impurities are expelled from the system.

5) The skin expels impurities that otherwise would have to be expelled by the excretory organs, and the skin is given a healthy glow.

In what ways can one exercise to receive the best benefits for restoration of the body to health? The most important results from exercise are realized when the exercise is in combination with the first two laws of health, sunshine and open air. Almost every time the Spirit of Prophecy mentions one of these laws, another is listed with it, if not both of them. "Outdoor life is the only remedy that many invalids need...How glad they would be to sit in the open air, rejoice in the sunshine, and breathe the fragrance of tree and flower...For those who are able to work, let some pleasant, easy employment be provided." *Ministry of Healing*, p. 264. Here all three aspects are listed as the most helpful remedies for the invalid.

Outdoor exercise best

What is the best exercise? "There is NO exercise that can take the place of walking. By it the circulation of the blood is greatly improved...Walking, in all cases where it is possible, is the best remedy for diseased bodies, because in this exercise ALL THE ORGANS OF THE BODY ARE BROUGHT INTO USE." *3 Testimonies*, p. 78. "A walk, even in winter, would be more beneficial to the health than all the medicine the doctors may prescribe...There will be increased vitality, which is so necessary to health." *2 Testimonies*, p. 529. "There is no exercise that will prove as beneficial to every part of the body as walking...Walking is also one of the most efficient remedies for the recovery of health of the invalid." *Healthful Living*, p. 130.

Walking is the best exercise

The other method of exercising that Heaven approves of is useful labor. In the world today people go to great lengths to get exercise. They participate in sports, go to gyms, invest in expensive machines, and many other things. But God has given us a guideline by which to know the proper, approved exercise. "Physical exercise in the direction of useful labor has a happy influence upon the mind, strengthens the muscles, improves the circulation, and gives the invalid the satisfaction of knowing how much he can endure." *Counsels on Health*, p. 199. "Useful labor that affords physical exercise will often have a more beneficial influence upon the mind, while at the same time it will strengthen the muscles, improve the circulation, and prove a powerful agent in the recovery of health." *Counsels on Health*, p. 627.

Exercise through useful labor

One last point to be made is stressing the importance of cardiopulmonary exercise. This is when the pulse rate is raised and kept up for at least twenty minutes. The safe level of the pulse rate is deter-

Cardiopulmonary exercise

mined by subtracting the person's age from 200. The pulse should not exceed this amount per minute to be on the safe side. Of course, an invalid, or sick person will not have the strength to achieve this at once. This is a goal to be worked toward that will give the most benefit to the entire system.

In the use of these three remedies—sunshine, open air, and exercise—healing will result. We can trust to God's Plan.

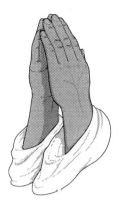

SIMPLE TRUST

Trust has been defined as placing confidence in or depending upon someone or something. In the complex ever changing world in which we live, people put their trust in many things. What should people trust in? Is there anything or anybody that can be trusted—completely trusted? Someone who is always the same—someone who is strong enough to deal with the toughest situation? Something that is absolute no matter where it is or what it encounters?

Who or what is to be trusted

The Bible tells us in *Hebrews* 13:8 that Jesus is the same yesterday, and today, and forever. Also, in *Malachi* 3:6 the Lord says, "I change not." The Bible, our guide book, tells us in whom we can trust and how to trust Him. *Proverbs* 3:4; "Trust in the Lord with all thine heart: and lean not unto thine own understanding. In all thy ways acknowledge Him, and He shall direct thy paths."

God does not change, neither do His laws. God has a plan for our health—eight simple laws. One of these eight laws that is often overlooked is trusting in God. Trusting not only that He will restore and preserve our health, but trusting also in Him in every area of our lives. "Thou will keep him in perfect peace, whose mind is stayed on thee: because he trusteth in thee." *Isaiah* 26:3. If the mind is kept on Jesus it will have peace. Peace of mind is a great contributing factor to maintaining or restoring health.

Peace result of trust in God

Worry, anxiety, discontent, depression, gloominess, all have a negative influence on the body. These kinds of emotions tend to break down our life forces by inhibiting the systems of the body to function properly and actually invite decay, disease, and death. Every cell in our body is affected by our emotions such as fear,

Lack of trust creates a negative influence on the body

hate, jealousy and anger. These emotions stimulate some organs while others are inhibited.

Stress

Today in society the term most often used to describe mental taxation is stress. Stress can be caused by many different situations: new job, divorce, financial troubles, and the everyday situations that all of us must face. Stress has become such a factor in the cause of sickness of people today that it is estimated that 70 to 80 percent of all illness is due to stress. To understand how this could be true it is necessary to realize what happens to the body when there is stress. Just what does stress do to the body?

Chemical reactions from stress

When the mind is made aware of something that is frightening, dangerous or even depressing it will send signals to the nervous system, in charge of hormones and other chemicals causing a negative reaction throughout the system. The adrenal gland receives a signal to release adrenalin. Adrenalin in turn will increase the heart rate and raise blood pressure sometimes causing a heart attack or stroke. Large amounts of blood sugar and oxygen are carried through the blood stream to the areas of the body that are directly involved in flight or fight situations. A high amount of adrenalin will cause the release of fats which clog the arteries, slowing the blood flow and eventually resulting in the heart being damaged. This is the physical result of great mental stress.

Other negative results

What happens when the mind is continually worrying? The result is not as quickly realized as with great fear or danger, but if the worry or stress continues for a length of time more damage will occur to the body. Some of the things that occur due to continual worry are: sodium retention which leads to high blood pressure, removal of proteins from cell structures which in turn cause wounds to heal slower. An increase of sodium results in potassium and hydrogen being flushed out of the system. Due to the decrease of potassium in each cell, the cells function less and less, and eventually die. The long term effect of cells dying eventually will effect the organs of the body.

Immune system affected

The immune system is affected by the stress on the mind. The immune system is strengthened by endorphin, a hormone secreted by the brain. The release of this hormone is reduced when stress occurs. Thus virus and even cancer cells can reproduce in the system.

The word of God has much to say on how mental attitude affects the health of the body. *Proverbs* 17:22 says, "a broken spirit drieth the bones." A broken spirit is one that is depressed, discouraged, etc. These emotions and others like them cause the bones to dry up. What effect does dried bones have on the body? The red blood cells carry the nutrients and oxygen through out the entire body. The red blood cells are made by the bone marrow of certain bones. If the bones dried up and did not produce the red blood cells, the body would not receive the nutrients or oxygen necessary for it to survive. Even some of the white blood cells, which are part of the immune system, are produced in the marrow of bones. Thus not only would the body not receive nutrients and oxygen, but the body would be greatly hindered in fighting infection if the bone marrow dried up. So we are enlightened in *Proverbs* 17:22, that "a merry heart doeth good like a medicine".

Attitude affects health

Calcium and phosphorus are both stored in the bones. Calcium is essential for many body functions, including strengthening the heart, soothing the nerves, and the vital role it plays in teeth and bones.

Proverbs 14:30 tells us: "A sound heart is the life of the flesh: but envy the rottenness of the bones." Often in the Bible, heart represents the mind. A sound mind is life to us while envy causes rottenness in our bones. Our attitude has a positive or a negative influence upon the body and the functions of the body, that is often times not realized.

Just as there is a negative reaction in the body due to stress, there is a positive reaction from trusting in God. Some of the positive responses that trust in God will promote in the body are:

Benefits received from trust in God

1) Cheerfulness promotes circulation and helps in the digestion process.
2) The will directed in the right direction will give energy to the nerves and soothe them.
3) The immune system is strengthened by trusting in God.

How can one learn to trust in God? Trust is developed in earthly situations by knowing someone and how they will react in certain situations. So it is with God, we must learn of His character to be able to trust Him. Faith or trusting comes from hearing the word of God. (*Romans* 10:17) To think on things that are true, honest, just,

Learning to trust God

pure, lovely, and of good report, (*Philippians* 4:8), will give peace of mind. To see God's goodness and love to everyone causes a response of trust. May each one look to Jesus and see His love, compassion, kindness, and concern for them alone and trust their lives to His wonderful plan for them.

Promises of peace of mind

"Come unto me, all ye that labour and are heavy laden, and I will give you rest. Take my yoke upon you, and learn of me; for I am meek and lowly in heart: and ye shall find rest unto your souls." *Matthew* 11:28, 29. God promises to keep our mind, *Philippians* 4:6, 7 tells us "to be anxious for nothing; but in every thing by prayer and supplication with thanksgiving let your requests be made known unto God. And the peace of God, which passeth all understanding, shall keep your hearts and minds through Christ Jesus." Won't you taste and see that the Lord is good today, and receive the peace of mind from God that is promised to all who will place their trust in Him. He has overcome the world, *John* 16:33, and has all power in heaven and earth, *Matthew* 28:18. Give your body the help it needs to get well or to stay healthy by trusting all to God.

(List below promises from the word of God that are special to you).

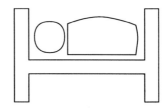

PROPER REST

In God's Plan, we have already studied sunshine, air, exercise and trust. In this lesson the benefits of rest or sleep will be studied. When a person exercises in the open air and sunshine the natural result will be fatigue. The cells in the body can not keep up their work indefinitely without rest. When one exercises, energy is used faster than it is restored; tissues are broken down faster than they are rebuilt; and poisons are formed faster than they can be eliminated. The body then needs rest to restore its cells, tissues, and organs to renewed vigor.

During sleep the body is repaired. All its activities lessen,—less heat is produced, the breathing is slower, the heart beats more slowly, digestion is lessened, the nerves and muscles are relaxed. The entire system is slowed down and the body building cells carry on their recuperative work. "They who sleep give nature time to build up and repair the weary waste of the organism." *Medical Ministry*, p. 80. "Sleep, nature's sweet restorer, invigorates the weary body, and prepares it for the next days duties." *1 Testimonies*, p. 395. Thus we understand that rest or sleep is essential for the system to be able to continue in its functions and also to build up the body.

Body repaired during sleep

There are several guidelines on how one should sleep to receive the greatest benefit.

Guidelines to receive the most benefit from rest

1) Have regular hours for sleep. By sleeping at regular hours every night, the health, spirits, memory and the disposition are improved. Irregular hours of sleeping cause the brain forces to be sapped.

2) Have an abundant supply of fresh air during sleep. Sore throats, lung diseases and liver disorders occur when there is not a continuous supply of fresh air during sleep. Also, one awakens feeling exhausted and feverish from the lack of oxygen. But, when there is a supply of fresh air while sleeping, a sound, sweet sleep is induced.

3) The stomach should have its work all done that it may rest as well as the other organs while sleeping. When the stomach is not empty before sleep the digestive process continues during the sleeping hours and this results in unpleasant dreams. Since the stomach has worked while you were sleeping you awake unrefreshed in the morning and with little desire for a hearty breakfast.

4) Early to bed and early to rise. The greatest amount of restoration is done to the body during deep sleep. Studies show that, due to the "circadian rhythm", which is regulated by the sun's rays, the deepest sleep occurs between 9 p.m. and 12 p.m.

Overwork double loss to system

"Nature will restore their vigor and strength in their sleeping hours, if her laws are not violated." *Healthful Living*, p. 69. When a person works two hours longer in the day than is best, the rest that the body needs is not received. Two hours of overwork plus two hours of lost sleep equals four hours of excess for the system. Also, the work done after normal work time is more taxing on the system and is most likely to be inferior in quality and quantity. In this way we are violating the laws of nature and the system is not fully restored to vigor and strength. The amount of sleep needed may vary according to the individual needs.

Needed for healing

When the body is sick in any way, it requires plenty of rest to heal. "She (patient) must have quiet and undisturbed rest." *Healthful Living*, p. 225. Mrs. White also tells us that the practice of sitting all night with the sick to watch them, is disturbing to their rest. This is especially true when two people stay with the patient and talk. She recommends that the caretaker be in another room, close to the patient, and respond to any calls for help. This would allow the patient to sleep undisturbed.

Inability to sleep

Often when one is sick it is hard to fall asleep. This is where the other remedies that have been studied in God's Plan are important. When enough exercise is received in the open air and sunshine, combined with a simple trust in God, sleep will be a natural occurrence. This is why all of God's Plan must be followed when restoring health to an individual.

Ways to obtain relief from insomnia

If there is still insomnia there are several natural ways that sleep may be induced. A neutral bath at a temperature of 94–97 degrees aids in reducing congestion of the brain and spinal cord. This frequently accompanies insomnia. When a person is very tired, nervous and worn out a fomentation (see appendix) to the spine will produce sleep. This should be applied very warm, not hot, for 20 to 30 minutes. The fomentation may also be given over the liver and stomach as well as the spine. Also, the following herbs are effective in producing sleep: Lady's slipper, catnip, skullcap and especially hops. Seep one teaspoon of any of these in one cup of boiling water for twenty minutes. Drink it when it is hot. These herbs are a tonic for the entire system and have no side effects as do sleeping pills. For some, a soothing massage releases the body of tension allowing a beneficial rest. Remember that hot and cold treatments are stimulating to the system and should not be used when trying to induce sleep.

Treatment for nervous exhaustion

"Tired nerves need rest and quiet instead of stimulation and overwork. Nature needs time to recuperate her exhausted energies." *Ministry of Healing*, p. 326. There is a treatment especially beneficial for nervous exhaustion. This is called the Wet Sheet Pack. It has three stages of effects on the system. The first is the cooling stage, 5–12 minutes, the body heat is removed by evaporation, this also reduces fevers. The second is the neutral stage, when the sheet is slightly warmer than the skin temperature—the amount of blood is lessened in the brain and sleep is the result. The third stage is the heating stage when sweating results in drawing blood from the congested organs. This treatment should not be used on someone with diabetes, severe colds, or one who is feeble or has skin eruptions.

The patient must be warm. Give the patient a hot foot bath for ten minutes, with a cold compress to the head. Have the patient void. Place the sheet in water that is 60–70 degrees and then wring it out. Wrap the patient in the sheet. They should be lying on a dry bed. Cover them with a blanket, allowing no air to reach the sheet. Leave for as long as necessary to obtain the desired result. This works great.

The combination of each part of God's Plan is necessary for the restoration of health to the body. May "every person have a knowledge of nature's remedial agencies and how to apply them. It is essential both to understand the principles involved in the treatment of the sick and to have a practical training that will enable one rightly to use this knowledge." *Ministry of Healing*, p. 127. May the knowledge learned in this lesson help all to fulfill the directions given in the statement above.

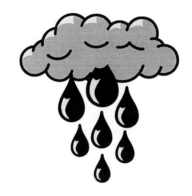

LOTS OF WATER

Water is one of the most abundantly supplied elements of nature. There is no other element of nature, with the exception of pure air, that is as important in sustaining life as pure water.

Necessary in sustaining life

The importance of receiving a fresh supply of water is understood when we realize the body is three-fourths water. The vital organs are all at least 70 per cent water. The blood and brain of the human body are composed of about four-fifths water. The fluid secretions (saliva, gastric juice, and liver bile, etc.) and excretions (skin perspiration and urine, etc.) are more than nine-tenths their weight in water, and these fluids need clean water regularly to perform their functions. Two-thirds of the body's water is found in the cells and the other one-third is outside the cells, either in the blood stream as plasma, in body cavities, or between the cells as tissue fluid.

The body is three-fourths water

Water is absolutely essential for the vital functions of the body to be performed. One system that is especially dependent upon water is the circulatory system. Water is the solvent which floats the blood corpuscles, nutrients, and waste elements which the blood is carrying. By the aid of water, nutrients enter the blood and are conveyed to fibers of the intricate human mechanism where repair and growth are needed.

Vital to blood stream

When water is taken into the system, it is received in the blood and increases the volume of the blood. This thinning of the blood quickens the circulation. When there is more blood, more water comes in contact with the waste matter and this waste matter is then more easily removed from the body.

Medium through which chemicals are transported

The body is full of many different chemicals. Each of these chemicals has a particular job in the regulation of the body's functions. Water is the medium through which these chemicals are transported to the various places in the system where they are needed to perform their duties.

Aids in digestion

Digested food is passed into the blood through the walls of the intestine, then from the blood these nutrients are passed into the individual cells. This process is then reversed. The wastes that each cell creates as a result of making energy passes from the cell to the blood and then on to the elimination points. Water is essential for this osmosis process to occur in the body.

Water also aids in other ways in the system. One example of this is when water in cooperation with chemicals breaks down the food in digestion and prepares it for absorption and use by the cells. The liver produces bile which aids in digestion by causing the fats to dissolve in water. If the body does not have enough water the fats cannot dissolve, resulting in a clogged system.

Note: while water aids in digestion we are to drink it one half hour before or two hours after a meal. Water should not be taken with a meal because it will retard digestion by diluting the digestive juices resulting in putrification of the food in the system.

Results of sufficient water

An abundant supply of water in the body results in the following:

1) All the moving parts are lubricated.

2) The blood is purified.

3) Organs in the body that are vital are invigorated.

4) The body temperature is regulated by water. (Without water, exercise would cause enough heat to coagulate the blood.)

5) Contributes to proper bowel elimination.

6) And aids in resisting diseases.

How much water is needed?

Just how much water does the system need every day? The organs of the body needs two quarts of water daily to function properly. Water is continually passing away from the body through the eliminating organs, such as the skin, kidneys, or lungs. The average person eliminates about five pints of water in twenty-four hours, and

80

an equal new supply must be replaced in order to preserve the fluidity of the blood.

Drinking water freely increases the function of the mucous membrane of the intestinal tract. This important organ of elimination when given plenty of water, passes more fluid on to the contents of the intestine. Thus ease of transit is increased helping with the universal trouble—constipation. This membrane also removes from the blood its foulest materials, rendering the blood cleaner for the building up of tissues. In this way water aids both in waste removal and tissue repair.

Aids in elimination

Even when not enough water is taken internally, the process of elimination continues. This robs water from the tissues and blood, and will hinder their ability to properly perform their much needed functions. The eliminating organs, the kidneys, skin, and lungs, when not supplied with enough water will be hindered in removing wastes from the system. These unremoved wastes will accumulate throughout the entire body clogging the system and causing an environment conducive to disease.

Lack of water

All of this has been dealing with water taken internally, but what benefit does the use of water externally give us? Baths do much more than simply clean the skin.

Uses of water externally

A warm bath soothes the nerves and equalizes the circulation. It also causes easier respiration, overcomes obstructions in the system. It is a benefit to the kidneys and urinary organs. The muscles become more flexible, the body and mind are invigorated, the intellect is made brighter and every faculty becomes livelier.

The above are especially true when a hot or warm bath is followed with an application of cool to cold water. It is not necessary that the water be so cold that the body is sent into shock, but there does need to be enough difference in the water temperature to cause the skin to react.

When used properly, external water can address the two limitations of the blood. The first limitation is that there may not be enough blood for an emergency need. External water treatments can, over a period of time, increase the amount of blood in the body. The sec-

Increase of circulation

ond limitation is the tendency of the blood to pool or congest in damaged or infected areas of the body. Hot and cold water applications will drain away the congestion of blood as well as bring a quantity of fresh newly-oxygenated blood to the area that needs it. Hot and cold water applications will also speed up the circulation of the blood.

The heart pumps the blood throughout the entire body, but in the more distant parts the heart cannot pump the blood along quickly. The blood vessels themselves have the ability to dilate and contract thus pushing the blood along. In reaction to applications of hot and cold water this dilating and contracting of the blood vessels greatly increases the circulation throughout the system.

Increases white blood and red blood cells

A hot water treatment followed by a cold water application increases the red blood cells from 20 to 35 percent. These red blood cells clean and nourish the body. But even more important, the white blood cells, which fight infections, are increased from 200 to 300 percent after a hot and cold water treatment. What a blessing these simple water treatments can be in the treatment of illnesses.

Effect of cold water treatment

The effect of a cold water treatment, temperature of the water below 85 degrees, is an instant contraction of the small arteries. If the cold application is prolonged, the area becomes bloodless. A brief application of cold water produces a momentary contraction followed by relaxation and an increase in the blood supply to the specific area.

Effect of hot water treatment

The effect of a hot water treatment, temperature of the water higher that 98 degrees, will increase the circulation. Hot baths are extremely stimulating to the system.

Effect of warm water treatment

The effects of a warm water treatment, temperature of the water between 85 and 92 degrees, are mild and soothing. The warm bath increases the action of the skin through absorption and perspiration.

Because water applied externally has all of these wonderful characteristics, we can identify the following healthful uses of water:

1) Toxins in the system are destroyed and the elimination of these toxins is increased.

2) Due to an increase in circulation and a stimulating effect on the eliminating organs, overall elimination is greatly increased.

3) Also due to an increase in circulation the body's metabolism and the formation of red and white blood cells is increased.

4) And there is relief from pain and nervous irritation.

It is easy to understand that water is one of heaven's choicest blessings after realizing all the ways that it contributes to the well-being of the body. Thank God for creating us so fearfully and wonderful and then providing us with the necessary gifts to keep the body in perfect health.

84

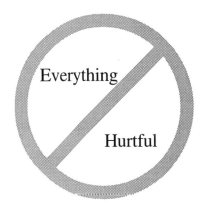

Everything / Hurtful

ALWAYS TEMPERATE

The eight laws of health are God's Plan for the restoring and maintaining of health in the human race. When looking at these eight laws the law of temperance seems unnecessary at times. But disregarding this law causes many consequences that greatly hinder the benefits received by observing the other seven. Understanding the true meaning of temperance and how it applies to the other seven laws is vital for God's Plan to work.

Must be combined with the other laws for health

Often in the society of today temperance is thought of as simply using or doing things in moderation. But this is not the definition given to us from Inspiration. The true definition of temperance that applies to God's Plan is given to us in *Patriarchs and Prophets*, p. 562: "True temperance teaches us to dispense entirely with everything hurtful and to use judiciously that which is healthful." Temperance in God's Plan is to dispense ENTIRELY with everything hurtful. There are many who have the attitude that some things will not hurt me if I only use them occasionally or in very small amounts. In God's Plan this concept will not work.

True definition

Not only are we to dispense entirely with everything hurtful, we are to use judiciously that which is healthful. The word judiciously means to "use good judgment, to be discriminating in the use of things". For an example of this consider: rest is good for us and necessary for health, but for one to sleep 18 to 20 hours a day would not be helpful for the system. Also, the elements necessary for the body to function must be eaten, but to overeat of any food, even if it is healthful, is not in keeping with this law of health and will overload the system causing many problems.

Applies to overall lifestyle

Often temperance is only thought of in relation to what we eat or drink. This should not, however, be the case as temperance applies to the entire lifestyle. Notice the following counsel given for us to have life abundantly: "In order to preserve health, temperance in all things is necessary,—temperance in labor, temperance in eating and drinking." *Healthful Living*, p. 68. "A strict compliance with the requirements of God is beneficial to the health of body and mind. In order to reach the highest standard of moral and intellectual attainments, it is necessary to seek wisdom and strength from God, and to OBSERVE STRICT TEMPERANCE IN ALL THE HABITS OF LIFE." *Counsels on Diets and Foods*, p. 32.

What are considered habits of life? Everything we do. The way we dress, drink, work, sleep, eat, study, exercise, etc. God has graciously given us counsel in all areas of our life so we do not have to guess as to what our habits should be.

Benefits gained from temperance

What are some of the benefits to be received by being temperant? The body will receive the necessary sun, oxygen, exercise, peace, rest, water, and nutrition. At the same time the body will not have to deal with an over abundance of any of these which would cause the system to not function properly. Notice the mental benefits that will be received from observing temperance in the following statement.

"The observance of temperance and regularity in all things has a wonderful power. It will do more than circumstances or natural endowments in promoting that sweetness and serenity of disposition which count so much in smoothing life's pathway. At the same time the power of self-control thus acquired will be found one of the most valuable of equipments for grappling successfully with the stern duties and realities that await every human being." *Education*, p. 206.

Must control the life of a Christian

"The law of temperance must control the life of every Christian. God is to be in all our thoughts; His glory is ever to be kept in view. We must break away from every influence that would captivate our thoughts and lead us from God. We are under sacred obligations to God so to govern our bodies and rule our appetites and passions that they will not lead us away from purity and holiness, or take our minds from the work God requires us to do. Read *Romans* 12:1." *Counsels on Health*, p. 42.

When following the eight laws of health it is essential to observe them all correctly. Temperance is the one law that holds the others together and insures that they will be observed in the correct manner.

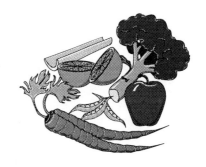

NUTRITION

The body is made up of cells and every cell has a specific duty that enables the system, as a whole, to function properly. The cells require oxygen, water, nutrients, and the prompt removal of wastes in order to maintain life. Nutrition is the act of providing the necessary nutrients for each different cell to properly perform its specific duty.

Providing necessary elements to cells

There are three classifications of foods essential for the cells of the body to operate properly.

1) Heat and energy foods which are made up of the starch, sugar, and fats that are eaten, commonly called carbohydrates.
2) The building and repair food which is protein.
3) And water, minerals, cellulose, and vitamins which regulate the body processes.

Three types of food essential for cells

These three groups all promote cell nutrition and cleansing. All disease is a result of improper cell nutrition and/or improper cell elimination.

Every cell needs energy to perform its individual function. All cells use amino acids and fatty acids combined with glucose and oxygen to make energy. Amino acids come from protein, fatty acids come from fats, while glucose comes from natural sugar found in fruits, etc., and oxygen from the air we breathe. These are essential elements for the proper function of the body. A proper amount of each element is essential. As in a car, if there is not the proper mixture of fuel, oxygen, compression, and spark, the engine will not run. So it is with the body. Each element must be received in the proper amount at the proper time to maintain health.

Cells require energy to function

Let us look at a few different aspects of the essential elements necessary to maintain life in the various cells.

Minerals essential

Elements that occur naturally in the earth such as iron, magnesium, phosphorus, and calcium are called minerals. Minerals are essential for the digestion of food. Minerals must be present in the system for food to be broken down and absorbed into the blood stream. The minerals are then used by the cells for energy. Minerals make up a large portion of all the digestive juices. When we do not get enough minerals in a well balanced diet to fulfill all the needs of the body, the digestive juices receive first priority. This means that the other parts of the body will have to go without the minerals they need in order to supply enough for the digestive juice. In this way disease, or an environment for disease, is created in the other parts of the body which lack the necessary minerals.

Minerals are essential in the contraction and relaxation of muscles. Calcium, sodium, and potassium in correct proportions are vital in all muscular movements. Minerals are important to all nerve cells. These nerve cells become irritated and nerve diseases develop as a result of insufficient minerals. The white blood cells, which constitute the majority of the immune system, require phosphorus to maintain their vigor. All of the glands require many different minerals to maintain their basic functions. (See glands) There are many other ways that minerals are used in the vital functions of the body, but from this you may understand the significance of receiving minerals in the diet.

Guidelines for receiving all elements needed

How can one receive the necessary minerals? There are some simple guidelines to follow to ensure that minerals, as well as all other necessary elements, may be obtained in the daily diet.

1) Eat raw foods. The eating of 60 to 80 percent of the daily diet raw will supply the necessary elements. When vegetables are cooked in water and the water is discarded from 10 to 70 percent of the minerals are lost.

2) Eat food unprocessed and as natural as possible. In the processing of foods most nutrient value has been removed.

Example

When wheat is refined into enriched white flour, the flour is devoid of almost all of its 14 nutrients including 87% of the fiber. This flour has been enriched to contain 4 of the 14 nutrients lost. The chart shows the percent lost of each of these 14 nutrients when wheat is refined into white flour.

PERCENTAGE OF LOSS IN REFINING WHEAT

B_1 ....86%
B_2 70
Niacin..86
Iron..84
B_6 60
Folic Acid..70
Pantothenic Acid..54
Biotin...90
Calcium...50
Phosphorus..78
Copper...75
Magnesium..72
Manganese 71
Food Fiber...87

Proper diet

What foods should be eaten to obtain a balanced diet that will provide the nutrients necessary to maintain abundant cell life? God outlined His plan for nutrition when man was created. In *Genesis* 1:29, God stated, "Every herb bearing seed... and every tree, ... which is the fruit of a tree yielding seed; to you it shall be for meat." This constitutes what man now calls fruits, nuts, and grains. After man sinned God added the vegetables to this diet. "And thou shalt eat the herb of the field." *Genesis* 3:18. Thus it is understood that the original diet for man, given direct from the Creator Himself, was fruit, nuts, grains, and vegetables.

Necessary nutrients in fruits, grains, vegetables, and nuts

The question is often raised, "Are all the necessary nutrients contained in these?" Ellen White has given counsel on this in *Ministry of Healing*, p. 296. "Grains, fruits, nuts, and vegetables constitute the diet chosen for us by our Creator. These foods prepared in as simple and natural a manner as possible, are the most healthful and nourishing. They impart a strength, a power of endurance, and a vigor of intellect, that are not afforded by a more complex and stimulating diet." And in *Counsels on Diet and Foods*, p. 92, "In grains, fruits, vegetables, and nuts are to be found ALL THE FOOD ELEMENTS THAT WE NEED." From these we learn that it is not necessary to eat from the animal kingdom to maintain a healthful diet.

Complex carbohydrates 80% of diet

The diet should consist of 80% complex carbohydrates, 10% fats, and 10% protein.

Fats 10% of diet

Protein to be from plant foods

a) Complex carbohydrates are those carbohydrates in a natural state, totally unrefined. Examples are all vegetables, grains, and fruit that are raw or just steamed.

b) Fats that are to be in this 10% are not free flowing or processed fats, but those that occur naturally in food. Examples of these are: avocados, nuts, olives, and seeds such as sunflower seeds etc.

c) Protein that is to be used is to be received from plant foods not animal derived. Examples of these types of foods are: beans, especially the soybean, peas, lentils, grains, seeds, and nuts.

In order to enjoy the benefits of proper nutrition in the system it is necessary for the stomach to be empty. Thus it is essential that five hours elapse between each meal. Not one bite of food should be taken between meals. The stomach also needs to be empty before sleep, in order that it may rest with the rest of the body. When the food is not digested before bedtime the sleep is disturbed, the brain and nerves are wearied, the whole system is unrefreshed, and is unready for the day's duties. In order to have the stomach emptied before sleep it may be best to eat only two meals per day. When these guidelines are followed the food eaten will not become fermented and the body will receive the proper nutrients for health.

When a person eats a balanced diet from the categories listed above, the cells will receive the proper elements to enable them to function properly. Thus the body will be in a state of health. God is so gracious to provide the many varieties of natural food for us. May we each eat of these freely and as a result have life more abundantly.

APPENDIXES

APPENDIX 1: EATING BETWEEN MEALS

It is a fact that eating between meals is not in the best interest of health. But do we understand why? What is the result of eating between meals on the body?

When food is eaten the stomach does its part of digesting this food and preparing it to move on to the small intestine. This process takes approximately three to five hours, depending upon the food that was eaten. When food is put in the stomach before it is completely emptied of the food from the previous meal, the whole digestion process must stop. The food that is partially digested must just wait in the stomach until the new food is digested to the same degree. The partially digested food will putrefy quickly in the warm, moist environment of the stomach. This waiting process causes the time before the stomach is empty and ready for the next meal to be much longer than normal.

Four nurses were given a normal breakfast of cereal, cream, bread and butter, a cooked fruit and one egg. In each case the stomach was empty when x-rayed in four hours. The next day this was repeated except that in two hours additional food was given with these results:

Nurse 1	ate one ice cream cone	6 hours after the meal the stomach was still at work
Nurse 2	ate nut butter sandwich	9 hours after the meal the food was still in the stomach
Nurse 3	ate one piece of pumpkin pie, glass of milk	9 hours after the meal some of the food was still in the stomach
Nurse 4	ate one banana	8 hours after the meal there was still food left in the stomach

In another study a nurse was given breakfast at 7:30 a.m. Four pieces of fudge were given during the day, one at 9:00 a.m., one at 11 a.m., one at 2:00 p.m., and one at 4:00 p.m. Dinner was eaten at twelve and supper at six. X-rays showed that nine hours after breakfast, the breakfast food was still in the stomach. Thirteen and one-half hours after breakfast the x-ray showed the breakfast food still in the stomach. The day before this study the breakfast food was digested in four hours.

Burden on entire system

A burden is placed on the entire system due to the fact that after this food has putrefied in the stomach it is passed on through the system and absorbed into the blood stream. Now that we understand what happens when we eat between meals, may we each, by the grace of God never eat between meals again and place this unnecessary burden on the stomach and the whole system.

APPENDIX 2: ALKALINE–ACID FOOD CHART

Alfalfa
Almonds
Apples
Apricots
Artichokes
Asparagus
Avocados
Bamboo shoots
Bananas
Beans, dried,
   green, lima
Beans, soy
Beans, string
Beets, fresh
Beet greens
Berries, all
Brazil nuts
Broccoli
Cabbage
Cantaloupe
Carrots
Carob
Cauliflower
Celery
Chard
Cherry juice
Citron
Coconuts
Collards
Cucumbers
Currants

Dandelion
Dates
Dill
Eggplant
Endive
Figs
Garbanzos
Garlic
Grapes
Grape juice
Grapefruit
Guava
Honey
Honeydew
Kale
Kohl-rabi
Leeks
Legumes, except
   lentils
Lettuce
Mangoes
Maple syrup
Milk, soy
Molasses
Melons, all
Mushrooms
Okra
Olives
Onions
Oranges

Orange juice
Papayas
Parsley
Parsnips
Peaches
Peas, dried, fresh
Pears
Peppers, green
Pineapple
Potatoes, all
Pumpkin
Radishes
Raisins
Rhubarb (oxalic
   acid)
Rutabagas
Sauerkraut (lemon
   only)
Soy beans
Spinach
Squash
Strawberries
Tomatoes
Tomato juice
Tangerines
Turnips and tops
Watercress
Water chestnut,
   fresh

Alkaline foods

Acid foods

Alcohol	Fowl	Mayonnaise
Barley	Frog legs	Oatmeal
Beef, all	Gelatin	Oysters
kinds	Goose	Peanuts
Bread, all	Haddock	Plums
Buckwheat	Halibut	Prune
Candy	Ham	Rice
Cheese, all	Hominy	Salmon
Cherries	Jams and	Shrimp
Chicken	jellies	Tapioca
Codfish	Flavorings	(starch)
Corn, canned	Lamb	Turkey
Cornmeal	Lentils	Veal
Coffee	Liver	Vinegar
Crackers,	Lobster	Walnuts
soda	Macaroni	Wheat
Eggs		

APPENDIX 3: HOT AND COLD FOMENTATIONS

A fomentation is when moist heat is applied to a specific part of the body surface. Fomentations are usually made of 50% wool to retain heat and 50% cotton to retain moisture. Towels may be used when fomentations are not available.

Fomentations

The effects caused by use of the fomentations are as follows:

1) Promotes an increase in the circulation of the white blood cells.
2) Causes an increase of blood flow to the skin, thus relieving internal congestion.
3) Relief of pain when used very hot for 3 to 5 minutes.
4) Soothing for nerves if moderate and prolonged—6 to 10 minutes—also for spasm of muscles or tension.
5) Increase toxin elimination by sweating.

Effects of fomentations

Fomentations are also excellent to induce sleep and for relieving chest congestion due to colds, bronchitis, etc.

Caution should be used in the following situations:

1) Do not use on legs or feet of diabetics.
2) Paralyzed or unconscious patient—due to danger of burning.
3) Patient who has heart problems or had a heart attack, place ice bag over heart before fomentations are laid on other body parts.
4) Stomach and bowel ulcers, and malignancy.

Cautions

There are three ways to heat a fomentation. They are as follows:

1) Boiling water

   Take a large bath towel, fold it lengthwise and place the middle two-thirds in a pan of boiling water. Twist the two dry ends to wring out the hot water. Place on skin or towel on patient's body.

2) Steaming

   Wet 5 large towels or fomentations and wring excess water out. Place in a large canner on the grid and steam for 20 minutes.

3) Microwave

   Wet and wring out towel or fomentation. Place in a large plastic trash bag. Put this in microwave for 4 minutes on high.

3 ways to heat fomentations

How to apply fomentations

To apply the fomentation to the patient, place the patient in bed and put feet in hot foot bath. Place one hot fomentation behind the patient's back. Then put a second fomentation on the chest area. Wait 4 minutes. Remove the chest fomentation and rub area with cold mitten friction. Apply another hot fomentation. Repeat this process 3 to 4 times. Cover the patient with a sheet and blanket at all times. If the fomentations or towels are wet or too hot, place a towel between the patient and the fomentation to protect the skin.

When the treatment is finished give the patient a cold mitten rub to cool the body. Dry patient with a dry towel and leave patient with completely dry garments and bedding. If these are even damp it will cause chilling and the benefits received from the fomentations will be lost. The patient then needs to rest in bed for the body to return to normal temperature and not become chilled.

APPENDIX 4: STEAM BATH

The following are effects that are the results of a steam bath:

1) Produces profuse sweating, releasing toxins

2) Opens up the sinuses, fights a cold, or influenza

3) Useful for rheumatoid arthritis

4) Increases, body temperature, pulse rate, blood pressure, and the body's metabolism

5) Prepares the patient for a cold treatment

Precautions:

The patient should be vigorous and basically healthy, not feeble. Use caution when giving this to a diabetic. Constantly watch the patient.

Equipment:

1) Straight chair, not metal as it will get hot and burn the patient

2) Hot plate, electric teapot, or electric skillet

3) Plastic tablecloth, shower curtain, etc.

4) Sheet and blanket

5) 3 towels—one on chair seat, one around neck, and one to turban hair (the last one is optional)

6) Ice bag—or wash cloth in ice water

7) Drinking water—not cold

8) Hot foot bath equipment

9) Oil of eucalyptus and peppermint if medicated steam is needed. Place drop or 2 of oil in water or rub body with the oil before the steam treatment begins.

Procedure:

1) Put hot plate under the chair. Place towel on the chair. Put container for hot foot bath in front of chair.

2) Seat the undressed patient and cover with the plastic. Place sheet and blanket over the plastic. Wrap the towel around the neck so no steam escapes.

3) Place ice bag on head or bathe the face with cold wash cloth constantly.

Effects of a steam bath

Precautions

Equipment for a steam bath

Procedure for a steam bath

4) Encourage drinking of warm water to induce sweating.

5) Check the pulse and temperature. Keep the pulse below 140 and the temperature below 104 degrees.

Rest half an hour

Give the patient a hot shower gradually reducing the water temperature to cool. Patient MUST rest in bed after the shower for at least ½ hour.

APPENDIX 5: VITAMINS

The body is made up of, and uses in its functions, the same elements that are in the dirt of the garden. There is one thing your body must have so that the elements the body receives from the food will be utilized by the system. Science has named this necessary ingredient 'vitamin'. The vitamin is the vital spark which vitalizes all the food elements and puts them to work. It is necessary for the growth of the body. The body may receive a generous supply of calcium, but without any vitamins the body can not use it in the formation of bones or teeth.

Necessary elements

Just what do vitamins do? It appears that they assist in the maintenance of every life process and the normal functions of every cell in the body. Some vitamins promote growth; others give health to the skin and glands throughout the body; some maintain nerve vitality; still others assist in building bones or aid in digestion, and so on through the whole system.

Assist in every life process

When vitamins were discovered they were named by letters of the alphabet such as A, B, C, and D, etc. Vitamins have always been present in the natural, raw foods. Everyone that science has found is present in either whole grains, vegetables, fruits, legumes, or nuts.

A brief look at some of the vitamins, their functions, and what foods they are most prevalent in, will help us to understand the important role they play in having good health.

Vitamin A maintains so many functions of the body they cannot all be listed here. One of the most important functions of vitamin A is the role it plays in the proper function of the glands. There are over 19 glands in the body that need vitamin A to function properly. There is evidence that the formation of kidney stones is prevented by vitamin A. Excellent sources of vitamin A are: kale, spinach, turnip tops, green lettuce, broccoli, green peas, green beans, apricots, prunes, and peaches. Some good sources are: avocados, cantaloupes, bananas, pineapples, dates, and orange juice.

Vitamin A

Vitamin B

This is a group of vitamins that are important to the metabolism of the body. The need of this group of vitamins is in direct proportion to the amount of carbohydrates that are eaten. A lack of B_1 or thiamin causes loss of appetite, loss of weight, lower body temperature and slowing of the heart rate. Also, when B_1 is deficient the nervous system is greatly affected. Excellent sources of B_1 or thiamin are: green lima beans, wheat germ, corn germ, wheat bran, oats, barley, brown rice, soybean, navy beans and dried peas. Good sources include: potatoes, sweet corn, cauliflower, beets, carrots, prunes, oranges, grapefruit, dates, apples, walnuts, almonds, and pecans.

Riboflavin or vitamin B_2

B_2 or riboflavin is important to the body in assimilating iron and proteins. It is water-soluble, so it is not easily stored in the body. A deficiency of B_2 or riboflavin causes loss of hair, skin disorders, and a general failure in physical well being. Excellent sources of riboflavin are: turnip tops, beet tops, mustard greens, soybeans, and the germ portion of wheat. Good sources include; lima beans, broccoli, cabbage, cauliflower, beets, carrots, lemons, grapefruit, pears, prunes, and peaches.

Niacin another B vitamin

Niacin, another B vitamin, works closely with proteins and amino acids for good health. The lack of niacin causes skin disorders, ulcers on the cheeks and lips, and a poor condition of the digestive system. Good to fair sources of niacin are: rice, green peas, turnip greens, soybeans, green cabbage, spinach, wheat germ, whole barley, and tomatoes.

Pyridoxine or vitamin B_6

B_6 or pyridoxine is helpful in the prevention of tooth decay, soothing of the nerves, and in maintaining the tone of the muscles. A lack of B_6 results in tension, insomnia, fatigue, irritability and weakness of the muscles. B_6 is found in cabbage, whole grains, brewer's yeast, and honey.

Vitamin B_{12}

B_{12} is a vitamin essential for the blood-forming organs of the bone marrow to function properly. It also helps to form hemoglobin, part of the red blood cells, and aids in the prevention of anemia.

B_{12} found other than in dairy products

Many are concerned about the total vegetarian getting enough B_{12}, as it is believed to be in animal products only. This should not be a concern if a balanced vegetarian diet is eaten, as B_{12} is definitely found in wheat germ, soybeans, and yeast. In *Counsels on Diet and Foods*, p. 313, we are told, "In the grains, fruits, vegetables, and nuts are to be found ALL THE FOOD ELEMENTS that we need."

104

On p. 322, of the same book it states, "The simple grains, fruits of the trees, vegetables, have ALL THE NUTRITIVE PROPERTIES necessary to make good blood."

Vitamin C

Vitamin C helps to form collagen, which holds the cells together in a wall of tissue. This aids in resisting infections. The nutrition and structure of the teeth are also affected by this. When vitamin C is lacking in the system, the joints become swollen and bones become porous and fragile. This is known as scurvy. Because vitamin C is destroyed in cooking and it is water-soluble, a liberal amount of raw food is necessary every day to receive the necessary amount of vitamin C. Excellent sources are: turnip greens, kale, parsley, spinach, sweet peppers, turnips, brussels sprouts, cauliflower, cabbage, broccoli, fresh and canned tomatoes, green peas, oranges, lemons, grapefruit, strawberries, cantaloupes, and sprouted seeds.

Vitamin D

Vitamin D aids in the absorption of calcium and phosphorus from the food. Vitamin D is created from a substance in the skin when the body is exposed to the sun's rays. Vitamin D sources have until lately, been thought to exist only in animal products. But, now it is known that vitamin D is present in canned string beans, raw spinach, raw carrots, corn germ, whole wheat, green cabbage, and fresh oranges.

Vitamin E

Vitamin E is valuable in maintaining normal red blood cells. It aids in tissue-building and is helpful for elasticity of the skin. Excellent to good sources are: lettuce, brown rice, barley, rye, wheat germ, lentils, nuts and the green leafy vegetables.

Vitamin F

Vitamin F promotes growth and is known as the unsaturated fatty acids. The unsaturated fatty acids combine with phosphorus to form a part of every cell. Vitamin F is valuable in preventing buildup of cholesterol in the arteries. A lack of this vitamin results in skin rashes, kidney disorders, and difficulty of wounds to heal. Sources of vitamin F are: olive oil, the avocado, and all nuts.

All vitamins in natural foods

All vitamins are always present in natural foods. Food needs to be eaten as a whole and in a good variety to receive the vitamins in a state that the body needs and can use. Also, when food is cooked with soda and baking powder the vitamins are killed. We can not use refined grains and then try to eat more fruits and vegetables to make up the loss. A BALANCED diet is essential to return to and maintain good health.

Index

A

Adrenal glands
    mineral, salt, and water balance regulated by, 41
    react to nervous system, 40
    regulates some metabolisms, 41
    secretes adrenalin, 40
    secretes cortisone, 41
Air, 63
    ionized, 64
    See oxygen
    purifies the blood, 6
    See oxygen
Alkaline
    food chart, 97
    reduces acid kidneys must eliminate, 35
    saliva, 11
Attitude
    affects health, 73
    positive or negative influence on body, 73
    proper, temperance aids, 86

B

Bile
    digests fats, 18, 25, 80
    digests fats-water aids in, 80
    produced by liver, 18, 25, 80
    stored in gallbladder, 25, 29
Bladder
    inflammation, 37, 38
    stores urine, 37
Blood
    carries wastes to eliminating organs, 1
    delivers nutrients, oxygen, and hormones, 1
    life of the flesh, 67
    purified by water, 80
Brain
    cerebral cortex, 51
    cerebrum, 51
    controls vital action of body, 52
    lack of blood results in stroke, 52
    needs glucose, 52
    needs oxygen, 52
    needs water, 52
    relationship to stomach, 52

C

Calcium
    essential for body functions, 73
    essential in teeth and bones, 73
    stored in bones, 73
    thyroid regulates level in blood, 40
    vitamin D aids in absorption of, 105
Carbohydrates, complex
    comprise 80% of diet, 91
    examples, 92
    metabolism of regulated by adrenal glands, 41
Carbon dioxide
    carried by red blood cells, 63
    waste residue from cell creating energy, 63
Cells
    four things they require, 63, 89
    make up body, 67
    require nourishment and cleansing, 68
    rquire energy to function, 67, 89
Cholesterol
    controlled by diet, 2
    damaging, available only from animal foods, 2
    definition of, 2
    high concentration of in eggs, 3
    increased due to improper bowel elimination, 3
    increased due to meat eating, 3
    increased due to saturated fats, 3
Circulation
    health depends upon perfect, 68
    heart circulates blood, 1
    increase of benefits body, 68
    increase of, list of benefits, 68
    sunlight increases, 58
    water increases, 79, 81
Colon, 19
    absorbs water and needed materials, 20
    delay of disposal-development of disease, 20
    disposes of waste, 20
    must be emptied for every meal eaten, 20
    putrification in burdens kidneys, 20
    putrification in burdens liver, 20
    putrification in burdens lungs, 20
    putrification in burdens skin, 20
    receives cellulose from small intestine, 19
    toxins absorbed into blood if not eliminated, 20

Other books by TEACH Services, Inc.

Absolutely Vegetarian *Lorine Tadej* ....$ 8.95
A complete guide to maintaining a strict vegetarian lifestyle. A way to reach your ideal weight and maintain it, as long as you live.

Activated Charcoal *David Cooney*...$ 7.95
This publication represents an attempt to gather together most of what has been reported to date on the use of activated charcoal as an oral antidote and as a remedy for other ailments.

Adam's Table *Reggi Burnett*...$ 8.95
A cookbook to help the user obtain optimum healthier and happier lifestyle through changes in their cooking style. Originated from Adam's Table Restaurant in Albuquerque, NM.

An Adventure in Cooking *Joanne Chitwood Nowack*...$12.95
This book has been compiled especially to teach young people, in a step-by-step, progressive way, the art of vegetarian cookery. Cooking is a real art, and very practical one too, since we need to eat every day.

Caring Kitchen Recipes *Gloria Lawson* $12.95
Specializes in recipes for better health that features: whole grains, vegetarian, dairy-free and nourishing dessert recipes.

The Celtic Church in Britain *Leslie Hardinge* ....$ 8.95
This is an authoritative study of the beliefs and practice of the Celtic Church which at the same time holds much interest for the non-specialist, containing as it does fascinating descriptions of the life of the early Celtic Christians in their monastic walled villages modelled on the Old Testament cities of refuge. Their elaborate penitential discipline was based on Old Testament compensatory regulations. Obedience to the Scriptures led them to establish a remarkable theocracy based on the laws of the Pentateuch and including the keeping of the Seventh-day Sabbath.

Champions of Christianity *Ronald C. Thompson*...$10.95
Champions of Christianity in Search of Truth will reveal the effects of the Counter Reformation against truth, including the efforts for truth undertaken by the Radical Reformation and the Great Revival.

Children's Bible Lessons *Bessie White* ....$ 3.95
These seven Children's Bible Lessons are prepared for use during Evangelistic Meetings, Bible seminars, Vacation Bible Schools, or at the Church's discretion.

Christian Faith & Religious Freedom *Olsen, V.N.* ....$ 8.95
The theological grounding provided in this book is an important antidote to the tendency of many to base their arguments on religious freedom and church/state issues on political or constitutional grounds. Dr. Olsen makes an important contribution to our thinking by making us face the theological bedrock of any Christian approach to these topics.

Convert's Catechism *Peter Geiermann*..$ 2.50
The quoted statement on changing solemnity from Saturday to Sunday can be found in this reproduction.

Cooking With Natural Foods I *Muriel Beltz*...$14.95
An ideal eating program for a preventive lifestyle, weight control and stress control. A program designed to give an alternative in the prevention and treatment of disease.

Country Life Natural Foods Something Better Cookbook...$14.95
This cookbook was originally designed to be used as a reference book in local community vegetarian cooking schools given across the country. Persons interested in better education in general health principles, and wholesome vegetarian recipes will find this cookbook a treasure to read, use and share. Completely revised and updated.

Divine Philosophy & Science of Health & Healing *G. Paulien* $19.95
All of the principles of the Bible and the Spirit of Prophecy are designed to allow us to function in perfect harmony with God Himself. This book discusses the methods and means of healthful living. It deals with going back to First Things, and relying by faith upon the substances which God has established for our benefit.

Don't Drink Your Milk *Frank Oski, MD* ....$ 7.95
Dr. Oski, the head of Pediatrics at Johns Hopkins University School of Medicine, gives the frightening new medical facts about the world's most overrated nutrient.

Earthly Life of Jesus *Ken LeBrun* $19.95
Biblical accounts of each event in Christ's earthly life carefully arranged together from the KJV Bible. Words of Jesus in red with full index.

Eden to Eden and Adam to Adam *Emilio B. Knechtle* ....$ 3.95
Originally published by Pacific Press Publishing Association, in 1890, this book is a most interesting study of the more important historic and prophetic portions of the Scriptures.

Garlic—Nature's Perfect Prescription *C. Gary Hullquist, MD* ....$ 9.95
Garlic, the Lily of Legend, has today become the focus of modern medical research. Recognized for thousands of years for its amazing curative powers, this bulb is today not only known for its potent bouquet but is drawing the attention of the scientific world as a potential antibiotic, anticancer, antioxidant, anti-aging, anti-inflammatory…the list goes on and on.

Gospel In Creation *E. J. Waggoner* ....$ 6.95
This book directs our wandering gaze to the open pages of God's created works as the expression of the gospel, the power of God to save from sin. Facsimile Reprint.

Grandma Whitney *Wm. Andress & Winnie Gohde*...$ 8.95
At 91, Hulda Crooks gained international acclaim by becoming the oldest woman to climb Mt. Fuji, Japan's tallest mountain. Six weeks later she broke her own record as the oldest person to climb Mt. Whitney. This is her story.

Healing By God's Natural Methods *Al. Wolfsen* ....$ 4.95
Al. Wolfsen has taught hundreds of sick people how to use only simple, non-poisonous remedies.

Healthful Living *Ellen G. White*...$10.95
Wherever this book has been received, it has been recognized as a veritable storehouse of seed thoughts relating to the great practical themes with which it deals. Facsimile Reprint.

Healthy Food Choices *Leona R. Alderson*...$14.95
Some special features include: guidelines for menu planning, breakfast suggestions, ideas for brown bag lunches, and much more!

Helps to Bible Study *J. L. Shuler*...$ 2.95
A Bible marking system which contains Bible studies covering twenty-eight topics including "The Second Coming," "The Seal of the Living God," "Bible Temperance," and "Christian in Dress." It is simple and practical in its approach, and will benefit all ages.

Hydrotherapy—Simple Treatments *Thomas/Dail* ....$ 8.95
Help your body overcome common diseases using hydrotherapy and simple home treatments.

Incredible Edibles *Eriann Hullquist* ....$ 7.95
Some "health" meals taste bland, some are hard to make, others require strange or hard to find ingredients. Eriann has developed a simple method of meal preparation where each recipe looks good and tastes great.

Mystical Medicine *Warren Peters* ....$ 7.95
Many people today have come to believe that our modern, technological system of health care in the Western world isn't proving to be the great boon that it was once thought to be. Frustrated and disillusioned people are turning to "more natural" methods of treatment. As we become aware of the intimate connection between the physical, mental and spiritual aspects of our nature, we are flocking to holistic medicine by the thousands.

Nature's Banquet *Living Springs* $12.95
Cooking is an Art and a Science. You will find that the art and science of cooking is especially enjoyable when using natural foods and when learning to be a vegetarian cook. The art of food preparation will give you the opportunity to exercise your enlightened preference and your personality to create attractive, delicious and nutritious meals. The science of cooking involves techniques and properties of food which affect its successful preparation.

Nutrition Workshop Guide   *Eriann Hullquist* .... 10 for $ 9.95

Chock full of nutritional recipes, as well as lots of helpful nutritional tips for special situations, such as road trips, fast foods, etc.

Quick-n-Easy Natural Recipes   *Lorrie Knutsen* ....$ 2.95

Every recipe has five or fewer ingredients and most take only minutes to prepare. Now you can enjoy simple, natural recipes without the drudgery!

Raw Food Treatment of Cancer   *Kristine Nolfi, MD*..$ 3.95

This book tells of the importance of raw vegetables in the diet of healing and general good health. Dr. Nolfi was a physician in Denmark for over 50 years.

Returning Back to Eden   *Betty-Ann Peters* ....$ 9.95

These recipes have been taste-tested by the world-wide travelers that have visited the Back to Eden Restaurant & Bakery in Minocqua, WI.

Steps To Christ Study Guide   *Gail Bremner*..$ 2.95

This study guide is designed to encourage the youth, and the young at heart, to understand and experience more fully a living relationship with Jesus.

Stress: Taming the Tyrant   *Richard Neil* ....$ 8.95

Stress is an inevitable part of our 20th century lifestyle. Under the proper circumstances stress can be uplifting as well as depressing. It can either help us grow our hasten or death. Find out how to control, manage and modify stress.

Swift Arrow   *Josephine Cunnington Edwards*...$ 8.95

A large family migrated over from Europe in the early 1700's and settled in Pennsylvania. After some time, one of the sons, Marcus Boylan, and his family decided to join others to travel and settle the frontier. Disaster struck when two young boys were stolen by Indians, one being Marcus' son George. This is a true account of his life with this Indian tribe, his eventual escape and journey back home.

375 Meatless Recipes–CENTURY 21   *Ethel Nelson, MD* ....$ 7.95

This book will help you learn how to feed your family in such a way that they will enjoy eating the foods that nutritionists tell us are an absolute must if we are going to make it into the twenty-first century.

Truth Triumphant   *B. G. Wilkinson* $12.95

The history of God's true Church from Ireland, to the Waldenses, the struggle to preserve the Bible and the pure doctrine of the apostles is disclosed. Facsimile Reprint.

Vegetarian Cooking School Cookbook   *Vierra* $11.95

Medical doctors and scientists are just now discovering a wealth of new facts about fruits and vegetables, and their findings are amazing. These foods contain high amounts of antioxidant nutrients and phytochemicals that not only nourish the body and build the immune system, but they prevent cancer...This unique cookbook contains over 170 of the tastiest vegetarian recipes as well as many facts and charts supporting why it is wise to avoid eating animal foods.

Who Killed Candida?   *Vicki Glassburn*..$17.95

Although diet is an important part of getting well, even the best food and supplements are undermined if you continue to unknowingly support yeast growth! The author will show you how making simple lifestyle choices can actually STOP THE YEAST SUPPORT CYCLE that other Candida programs do not address.

Whole Foods For Whole People   *Lucy Fuller*...$10.95

Whole Foods For Whole People is not just a cookbook, but a manual to teach people how they can live a longer, healthier lifestyle by using the natural resources which surround us.

To order any of the above titles, see your local bookstore.
However, if you are unable to locate any title,
call 800/673-3742